CHILDHOOD
ILLNESS

CHILDHOOD ILLNESS

A Common Sense Approach

JACK G. SHILLER, M.D.

Illustrations by Neil O. Hardy

STEIN AND DAY / *Publishers* / New York

First published in 1972
Copyright © 1972 by Jack G. Shiller
Library of Congress Catalog Card No. 71-186817
All rights reserved
Published simultaneously in Canada by Saunders of Toronto, Ltd.
Designed by Bernard Schleifer
Printed in the United States of America
Stein and Day/*Publishers*/7 East 48 Street, New York, N.Y. 10017
ISBN 0-8128-1460-6

FOURTH PRINTING, 1973

To Doris
who asked all the questions
and
to Beth, Steve, and Andy
whom the questions were all about

Contents

Introduction

I am a pediatrician. I have a busy practice, I enjoy my work, and I count most of my patients' parents as my friends. Nevertheless, my mothers would like to avoid me. Specifically, they would like to avoid bringing their children into the office for minimal illness or for problems they think they ought to be able to manage at home.

But they don't know how. They often can't differentiate major from minor illness, and so they worry about it. The mass media have bombarded them with discoveries of horrendous diseases and they don't want to neglect their children's health. On the other hand, they don't want to waste a doctor's time, and they don't want unnecessary medical bills. So they're hung up on the horns of a dilemma, and they struggle. But the struggle is usually short-lived. After all, it's better to be safe than sorry, and no one can criticize a mother for being concerned about her child's health. So they continue to come to the office.

Sometimes they come right out and ask, "How can I

know when to call?" I get the feeling that they're really asking me how to know when *not* to call. But this is not what they say. After an office visit in which no specific medication has been prescribed, they are more likely to indicate their frustration with parting remarks like "Just wanted to be sure," or "Well, I feel better now that you've seen her," or "Sorry to bother you."

What comes across to me is that the mother is either berating herself for spending the price of an office visit needlessly, or feeling guilty because she thinks she has wasted my time.

Let's take a closer look at the genesis of these feelings. Where do modern mothers learn their *mothercraft* anyhow? Time was when child care was handed down from mother to daughter through successive generations. There was always an older, experienced female relative on hand to provide on-the-job training. But after the Second World War, millions of new sets of parents were created amid a mass upheaval of the population and the ensuing destruction of large-family units. The urban movement completed the disruption, and when the baby boom came in the middle and late forties, grandparents usually weren't around to tell new mothers what to do.

But Benjamin Spock was, and he did a masterful job. Postwar generations of mothers followed his book like a catechism, and their children thrived. The void was filled, and mothercraft was saved. Almost.

Spock's forte was child development. He had a year of psychiatric training before he opened a practice and, following the success of his book, left that practice to work full time in child psychiatry and development. That was in 1947. It is interesting to note that of the more than five hundred pages in Spock's original hard-cover volume, fewer than one hundred were devoted to sick children. Even the new, revised paperback edition, published in 1968, has approximately the same proportions. Most of the book dealt with special problems of infancy; the normal child at various ages; child development, behavior, nutrition, and routine care. And because he is a physician of great dedication, in the section on children's diseases he carefully cautioned his readers to call the physician at very safe stages in the progression of their children's illness.

Meanwhile modern medical miracles were taking place with amazing rapidity, and they did *not* lend themselves to do-it-yourself application. The body was still sacred to the physician, and no one trampled on hallowed ground. Nevertheless, anything having to do with child care makes good copy, and announcements of new medical developments were promptly publicized for maternal consumption. Most of them contained dire warnings of catastrophe in the event of neglect.

Enter the era of panic pediatrics.

The pediatrician, who, in treating children, had been competing with the general practitioner, now found his services more and more in demand. In the child-oriented world of the fifties and sixties, mothers took their children to the pediatrician in sickness and in health, and, in so doing, gave up more of their mothercraft. It was so much easier to let the doctor do the worrying, and he was happy to—for a fee. Minimal-illness visits became commonplace, and the doctor's bill became a well-established part of the monthly family budget.

But what of the seventies? What are a mother's needs now, after twenty-five years, hundreds of baby books, and all the modern miracles? I believe that mothers are ready to have some of the panic taken out of pediatrics. They want to know what *not* to worry about as well as what *should* concern them. They want to be able to differentiate well children from sick children, serious illness from trivial illness. More specifically, they want to know when and when not to call the doctor. One might say they are ready for "do-it-yourself pediatrics." Very few, if any, of the current child-care manuals emphasize illness or common physical problems. Here, I think, lies the need.

Many conditions that are still described in the current literature have become insignificant compared with some of the major problems now with us. Consider polio. In 1951, this disease killed or crippled thirty-six thousand children. Now, with vaccine, doctors see fewer than fifty cases a year nationwide. Statistically this puts polio in the same category as bubonic plague.

Conversely, we now recognize problems that were hardly thought of, much less written about, twenty-five years ago. Look at nutrition. The importance of vitamins and warnings of deficiency diseases still appear in baby books. But I've been in practice for fifteen years and have yet to encounter a case of rickets or scurvy. The *mal*nutrition that I see day after day is obesity. Fortunately, I don't follow these children into adult life and don't have to treat the hypertension, high cholesterol levels, and coronary artery disease that result. This is one example of a traditional aspect of pediatrics that needs new emphasis.

There are also practical reasons for writing this book. The population grows by leaps and bounds; everyone agrees that the production of doctors cannot and will not keep up with population demands. Fewer doctors declare their intention of specializing in pediatrics every year. At the same time, the average age of the population is declining. In

1980, 50 percent of the population will be younger than twenty-one years of age!

Who is going to take care of all these children? Pediatricians are now talking about assistants in practice, specially trained (beyond nursing) personnel to help the pediatrician by performing technical procedures and less complicated medical tasks. I am not sure this is the answer. In addition, assistants have to be paid, which adds another dimension to the high cost of medical care.

I believe the best answer is fewer visits to the pediatrician's office. If this is to be achieved, young mothers need a better basis for evaluating their children's illnesses and need to be able to trust this evaluation. Often much of the problem can be alleviated with a "tincture of time" and some "judicious neglect." These prescriptions indeed can be dispensed in many instances, thus saving much of the pediatrician's time and the family's medical dollar.

My purpose, therefore, in writing a book about common childhood illness is three-fold: to indicate when simple disease can be treated at home; to alert parents as to when competent professional medical help should be sought; and to enable young mothers to take better care of their sick children.

I have *not* dealt with psychological, emotional, or developmental problems because these subjects have been exhaustively treated in other volumes by people with the training to write about them. And I have *not* dealt with accidents and injuries, because those subjects alone demand a whole volume. Including them here would change the character of this book, which is about illness.

On the other hand, the extensive explanations of the mechanisms of certain diseases that appear in this volume have been prompted by the number of questions about them that have been put to me by inquisitive parents. I have noticed that the level of cooperation in treatment is much higher when parents know *why* they have been instructed to do something. Further, a basic understanding of the mechanism of an illness that may occur can help parents initiate home remedies that work.

A word of caution. I am not advocating minimal medical care for children. Modern medicine has much to offer our children in the way of prevention and cure of disease, the alleviation of symptoms, and the enhancement of a general state of physical well-being. Periodic checkups are important, especially in the early years, and should be continued throughout life. Immunizations are a must. Many childhood diseases are completely preventable.

Many sick children *should* be seen by their physicians—some sooner and some later—to cure the disease, make them more comfortable, prevent recurrence, and forestall complications. It is my purpose here to make available to parents guidelines for deciding when a child needs the doctor's help.

In Part I, the chapters are arranged by symptom complex rather than by age group or body part. Their sequence has been determined by how often the complaint has been made to me in my experience as a pediatrician. My intention is to give you the information you are most likely to require first.

Part II attempts to explain some uncommon illnesses and other terms which do not relate to the body of the text, but about which you may have questions. An appendix of standard information is also included which supplements the text and provides additional information regarding immunizations, drugs, growth charts, and so on. All of this information is indexed.

Finally, my thanks to David Oliphant, who encouraged and sustained me; Roberta Maltese, who helped me with the manuscript; my professors Rustin McIntosh and William A. Silverman, who reassured me; Neil Hardy and Jan White, whose illustrations and chart design illuminated the text; Boyd Givan and Dave Friedman, who helped me with the section on ethical drugs; and all the editorial staff at Stein and Day, who took a manuscript and made a book out of it.

PART I

1

The Suddenly Ill Child

The child is not the little man. This is perhaps the cardinal principle upon which the specialty of pediatrics is founded. Children are physically different from adults in many ways other than size, and not knowing how they differ is what makes for the uncertainty, confusion, and even panic that arise in caring for sick children. First of all, if they're small enough, they can't tell you what hurts them. And when you know they're in pain but don't know why, that's pretty scary. Secondly, children get sick fast— faster than adults. As a matter of fact, biologically they do everything faster than adults. They breathe faster, have faster heart rates, consume proportionately more calories in a day, and require more water pound for pound than adults. The compensating feature here is that they get well faster, too.

Children are really pretty resilient. They get sick and get well, and they seem to do both quite easily. So, the object of the game is to learn to decide which illnesses you have to worry about and which ones you don't. For this reason I want to discuss the seriously ill child first, the child who has symptoms that you need to recognize and deal with promptly. Let's face it, you're over your head as far as the care and treatment of this child are concerned, and you want to seek competent professional help quickly. But first you have to recognize that he's *really* ill.

You must first decide whether any of the following vital functions is being impaired:

State of consciousness. Has the child's state of consciousness changed? Is he almost unconscious? Is he delirious? Does he slip back and forth between being lucid and not making sense?

Respiratory distress. Is he having *serious* trouble breathing? Is his color bad—pale or bluish—because he's having trouble getting air?

Fluid intake and output. Is he drinking liquids? Is he vomiting? Is he urinating? How much? I am not talking about the child who vomits once or the infant who wakes up for the first time with a dry diaper. I'm talking about the child who has vomited several times, or has not voided in twenty-four hours. Such deviations from the normal are significant enough to be brought to the attention of your physician.

Most often when a child has fever, it means he has an infection. Most often when he has an infection, it is viral. And most often if he has a virus, antibiotics won't help it. You should call the doctor if your child experiences severe disturbances of the vital functions: state of consciousness, respiratory distress, or fluid intake and output. If these functions are not being impaired, you can usually take the time to wait and see.

After that you need to know how to care for the less seriously ill child. You should know how you can tell when a child is sick, what fever means, how to recognize specific symptoms, and how to use medication correctly. You will also need some general hints on caring for a sick child. Remember that this is an introductory, general chapter on how to think about sick children and how to try to appraise their condition. Later chapters will deal more specifically with diagnosis and treatment. But here you will learn how to recognize and deal with problems promptly, and which of them you can handle yourself. Let's try to take some of the panic out of pediatrics and bring back the common sense our parents used.

THE SICK CHILD: GENERAL BEHAVIOR

The first sign that a child is sick is a change in behavior. The change may be subtle or dramatic, but it is always present. Behavioral changes usually occur in relation to three different areas: the child's usual self; age-group differences, and the expected degree of abnormality.

The Child's Usual Self

Show me a toddler who falls asleep while playing at the beach, *never before having fallen asleep while playing at the beach,* and I'll bet he has a fever when he gets home. When the infant with a voracious appetite stops eating for more than one to two feedings, something is wrong. When the eight- to nine-year-old hellion starts lying around the house after school, he's got a problem. These are all examples of children departing from their usual routines, any of which may be the first sign of illness.

Age-group Differences

The three examples just given also illustrate age-group differences that must be considered. What behavior is appropriate to what age group? The newborn spends most of his time sleeping; the older child who spends most of his time sleeping has a problem. The toddler's mood swings wildly from happiness to tears and tantrums in minutes, back and forth, many times during the day; the adolescent who does this shows markedly abnormal behavior that may signify serious mental or physical disorder. The four-year-old girl with a bloody vaginal discharge has a medical problem requiring careful investigation; the twelve-year-old girl with the same symptom is probably having her first menstrual period.

Behavior More Abnormal Than Usual

The most difficult differences in symptoms to pick up, and the most subtle ones, are deviations from a "predictable" abnormality in any situation. Let's take the child who has chicken pox. He is *expected* to run a low-grade fever, have pox that itch and scab, and generally not be very sick. But if this child has high fever for more than a day or two, develops a bad cough, or complains of severe headache, you should recognize that his behavior has now become *unusual* for chicken pox, and seek help. Similarly, infants who spit up don't usually have diarrhea (when they do, gastroenteritis or food intolerance is more likely); toddlers who have "colds" don't usually cry all night (bet on an earache); and adolescents who are more tired than usual when they have routine sore throats and swollen glands may have infectious mononucleosis.

Specific Symptoms

If you are lucky and your child is old enough, he'll tell you exactly what is wrong with him. Earache, sore throat, and congested cough are examples of complaints that, when associated with fever, usually mean infection in the area of the complaint. (These are also the obvious ones; their treatment will be discussed in Chapters 2 and 3.)

Sometimes the child's complaint involves whole functional systems. Vomiting and diarrhea point to the gastrointestinal system. Cough, chest pain, wheezing, and nasal obstruction involve the respiratory tract. These symptoms indicate systemic infections that may produce fever.

An important consideration is knowing the child. If an infant or toddler has had an ear infection in the past and he gets up at night, obviously in pain, with fever and a cold, he can be assumed to have another ear infection until proven otherwise. Interestingly, this child may not be able to localize his discomfort. Many children are brought to my office complaining of bellyache when their real problem is a red-hot ear. On the other hand, the child who is known to be allergic and who begins sneezing when he gets into the country for a Labor Day picnic (hay fever season) is probably not coming down with a cold. Check the pollen count.

FEVER

It has been said that fever is only a symptom, and as such may even be a friend. As recently as fifty years ago, fever therapy was used successfully in the treatment of many diseases. Eye ailments and disorders of the nervous system were treated with injections of dead typhoid bacteria that produced fevers of up to 107° F. Some of the more recent medical literature describes a substance called *interferon,* which is released by the body to fight viral infection and is more effective at higher temperatures (that is, while the patient has a fever).

We therefore need to take a new look at fever: is it good or bad, normal or abnormal? Should it be treated or not?

Normal Variations

The first normal variation that must be considered is that of the thermometer. The manufacturer's warranty notwithstanding (he is liable only as far as replacement is concerned), good clinical thermometers have been found to vary from .4° to .6° F. Therefore, when you are taking comparative temperatures (that is, morning and night), you should use the same thermometer.

Rectal temperatures are usually .6° F. higher than oral temperatures, which are usually 1° F. higher than armpit temperatures. Instead of remembering which is higher or lower, and by how much, simply use the same anatomical location each time so that the readings will be comparable.

Temperatures also vary according to time of day (see Figure 1), temperature of the environment, and degree of activity just prior to having one's temperature taken.

A child sleeping in a cold room can have a *rectal* temperature of 97° F. An adolescent exercising vigorously on a hot summer day can be measured at 103.5° F. *orally.* Remember that many factors can play a role in a temperature measurement.

Perhaps the biggest villain in the temperature game is that little arrow pointing to 98.6° F., which implies that

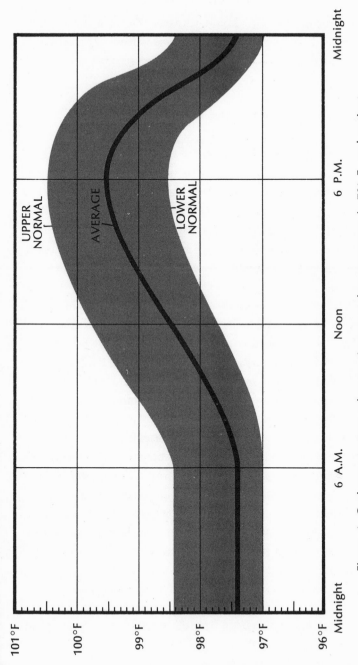

Figure 1. Oral temperature when environmental temperature is 70° F. and patient has been resting ten minutes before measurement

every normal person should measure that temperature all the time at any part of the body. This is not only impossible but absurd.

How and Where to Take the Temperature

Generally speaking, I am for taking rectal temperatures most of the time. The rectal method is fast and accurate. The armpit method is less reliable, and the oral method is usually worthless for a child under eight years old. Most children whose temperatures need taking have upper respiratory infections. They can't breathe through their noses. They keep their mouths open, and the oral reading is worthless.

The only difference between oral and rectal thermometers is in the bulb. The oral thermometer has a greater surface area than the rectal, whose bulb is shorter and gently rounded. *With care* they can be used interchangeably. The rectal thermometer will measure oral temperatures satisfactorily if it is left in for a full three minutes and if the child's mouth is kept closed. An oral thermometer can be used in the rectum if it is lubricated and if the child is old enough and cooperative. Because of the danger of perforating the rectal wall, the oral thermometer should *not* be used in this way with younger or struggling children.

Thermometers should be well wiped with alcohol after each use. During the few days that a child may be ill, it is also a good idea to let the thermometer sit in alcohol between uses.

A good technique for taking the rectal temperature of an infant or uncooperative toddler (see Figure 2) is to place the child on a table, bed, or your lap, with his bottom

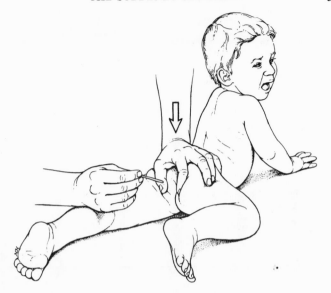

Figure 2. How to take a rectal temperature

up. You can immobilize him by placing the heel of your other hand in the small of his back and pushing down. Don't let him get his knees under him. If he does, you've lost the round. With the thumb and index finger of the same hand, spread his buttocks, and you will be able to insert the thermometer easily with your free hand. With the child in this position and the thermometer one third to one half of the way in, you can read the temperature while it is being measured. You will see it move up rapidly; when it stops moving, remove the thermometer.

Chills and Fever: The Human Thermostat

The first sign that a child is developing fever often will be his complaint that he is cold. But if you measure his

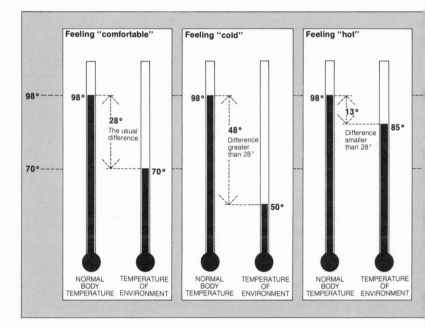

Figure 3. The human thermostat

temperature, you will find it elevated. Why then does he complain of being cold? To understand why, you need to understand the human thermostat.

We have learned to sense comfort by maintaining a usual *difference* between our own body temperature and the temperature of the environment. This comfort zone is usually an environmental temperature 28° F. lower than normal body temperature. Thus, 98° F. *minus* 28° F. equals 70° F., which is comfortable. (These figures are approximate.)

In cooler weather, the body-environment difference is *increased* (because of the lower environmental temperature, for example, 55° F.). Thus, the difference has increased to 43° F. We have learned to associate such a change with

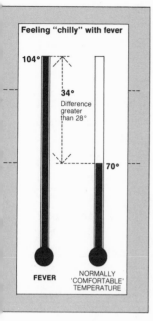

Feeling "chilly" with fever

104°

34°

Difference greater than 28°

70°

FEVER

NORMALLY 'COMFORTABLE' TEMPERATURE

being cold. In warm weather, the usual difference is *decreased* (because of the higher environmental temperature, for example, 85° F.). Now the difference has decreased to only 13° F. We have learned to associate this change with being warm. (See Figure 3.)

All these changes have occurred because the temperature of the environment has varied while the body temperature has remained constant. But if the body temperature varies while the temperature of environment remains constant, the same net effect can occur and our previously learned associations trip us up. For example, if the body temperature is elevated to 104° F., the difference has increased, and past experience tells us that we ought to be cold! The chills are real, even though the change in environmental temperature is not.

Let's look at what's really going on. Infection produces fever in a number of ways. The battle between cells and bacteria (or viruses) causes their destruction, and toxic breakdown products, or pyrogens (substances that produce fever), are released. In addition, increased metabolism during infection causes the body to use a greater number of calories. This, in turn, causes the body to use more water, which results in a mild dehydration and fever.

Getting back to the body thermostat, pyrogens increase the setting of the thermostat, calling for more heat. Chills therefore are produced to generate that heat. The thermostat may be reset by administering aspirin (doctors don't know how this works, but it does), or by bringing the fever down in other ways.

Significance of Fever: Infection and Viruses

There are two primary questions that should be asked about infection: Where is it? Is it bacterial or viral? Leaving the first question to the section in this chapter on Specific Symptoms, let's look at the type of infection.

According to various estimates, 75 to 90 percent of all childhood respiratory infections are caused by viruses. Antibiotics and chemotherapeutic agents do not as a rule combat viruses, although there are some rare exceptions. Yet antibiotics are prescribed (needlessly) for well over three quarters of all sick children.

The fault lies partially with the mother, but more so with some physicians. From the physician's point of view, when he prescribes antibiotics he needs to worry less about the accuracy of his diagnosis ("If it's not a virus, then the antibiotic will probably take care of it"). And then, when the child's temperature goes up at night, the mother won't call the physician in a panic because "now the child is sicker and needs an antibiotic." Fallacious reasoning, of course, but it's sometimes easier to prescribe than to argue.

There is often a tremendous amount of parental pressure put upon physicians for the shot of penicillin to "get it faster," "nip it in the bud," "prevent secondary bacterial infection," and so on. This is just not so; such reasoning has been proved false time after time.

On the other hand, why not prescribe the antibiotic? Why not be sure? There are two very good reasons. Many antibiotics have harmful side effects and, in certain patients, can produce unusual reactions (drug idiosyncrasies) that are usually more difficult to treat and cure than the original disease. In addition, there is evidence that the treatment of viral diseases with antibiotics may actually make the diseases worse. Even more important, doctors are very anxious that children should *not* become allergic to the agents most effective in treating several bacterial infections.

Flu and grippe symptoms—fever, achiness, runny nose, scratchy throat, slightly upset stomach, tiredness, malaise ("I just don't feel good"), headaches, or any combination of a number of these symptoms—usually mean viral infection. One almost certain symptom of flu or grippe is achy eyes. All these symptoms respond to the tried and true remedies of aspirin, bed rest, and lots of liquids.

My own prescriptions also usually include that "tincture of time" and some "judicious neglect." Most visits to the pediatrician can be avoided if the mother will just take a little time to wait and see—unless the child is seriously ill.

Convulsions

Most children will never have a convulsion—even with a temperature of 105° F. But a few will, and if it happens to be your child, your statistics have just jumped to 100 percent.

The younger the child and the higher the temperature, the more apt he is to have a febrile convulsion. Roseola is more commonly associated with febrile convulsions than any other childhood illness. They are most apt to occur in an infant or toddler with very high fever who is noticeably irritable or begins trembling. Suddenly he will stiffen out and the eyes will roll back in his head. If he is sitting up, the stiffening out process will make him appear to have thrown his head back. His fists will clench, elbows and

knees will flex, jaws will be clamped together, he will sali-
vate, hold his breath and turn a little blue. Urine and/or
feces will frequently be lost. The convulsion is usually brief
(seconds to minutes). The very small child will "awaken"
and begin to cry. If he is slightly older and hasn't been
panicked by the adults around him, he will wonder what
happened and then want to go back to sleep. Sleep is okay
here; he will awake in an hour or so feeling much refreshed.
But he must be cooled off first!

In general and pediatric practices, febrile convulsions
—convulsions that occur with fever—are fairly common.
(This is not to say that they are not important.) They are
generally harmless disturbances of the central nervous system and, when properly controlled, are not usually followed
by any permanent damage or aftereffects. When dealt with
promptly and correctly, their treatment is satisfactory, recurrence can be prevented, and the child outgrows them
within a few years.

There are things we still do not know about febrile convulsions: Why do they occur at all? Why do some children
get them with fevers of 103° F. when others do not with
fevers of 105° F.? Are they related to how high the fever
goes or to how fast it gets up there?

But the fact is, febrile convulsions do· occur, and the
first time around parents are not prepared. Because the
convulsions are associated with fever, the typical response
of those who lack more specific know-how or medicine is
to try to bring the fever down. This is exactly right. But
first, *call the doctor.* Two out of three of the criteria of
critical illness are present in this situation: The child is
unconscious, and he is having trouble breathing.

You must try to establish an airway. Be sure that the
child's nose is clear and/or his mouth is open. Insert some

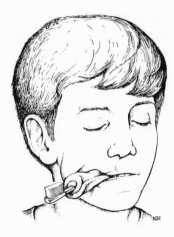

Figure 4. The use of a blunt object such as a toothbrush in convulsions

blunt object (such as a toothbrush handle) wrapped in a handkerchief between his upper and lower back teeth on one side (see Figure 4). This will keep him from biting his tongue.

It makes no sense to try to give aspirin to a child who is having a convulsion. Aspirin suppositories are available over the counter and should be kept in the refrigerator for use in place of aspirin tablets. Use half a five-grain suppository for infants under two years, a whole one for the two- to four-year age group, one and a half for the four- to six-year-olds, and two whole suppositories for a child over six. (There are also ten-grain suppositories available for older children.)

Whether you have a suppository on hand or not, it makes sense to get the child cooled off fast. This means you will have to use cool water (in or out of the tub), ice packs, rubbing alcohol, a cool room, and/or a fan *imme-*

diately. All these methods work. *Don't* warm the child when he starts to shiver and develop goose bumps. That just means he is cooling off rapidly, which is exactly what you want. His natural body defenses against lower temperatures are beginning to work. Take his temperature, and if it is still in the 104° F. range, keep up the cooling until it is down to a respectable 102° F. And don't forget the aspirin. Remember that the body thermostat needs resetting.

Having done the job, don't ruin it by adding flannel pajamas, blankets, and the heating pad. If you do, his temperature will be back up to 105° F. before you get the light turned off. Let him wear light pajamas or just underwear, and cover him with a sheet. He will be much more comfortable after a while, and so will you.

Your doctor may want to prescribe medication for this or future episodes. And he will want to give you additional instructions. Sedative drugs such as phenobarbital may be in order—at least until the child is five or six, the age at which most children outgrow their febrile convulsions.

Essentially there are two schools of thought regarding the administration of sedatives to a child who has febrile convulsions. Some doctors feel that rapid-onset fever, which is frequently unpredictable, requires daily preventive medication throughout the toddler years. Most children who receive daily sedative medication for the prevention of convulsions tolerate these low doses very well; the medicine does not appear to affect their activity or alertness. Other doctors feel that sedative medication and aspirin should be given concurrently in the treatment of fever and that most febrile convulsions can be prevented in this way, without resorting to daily medication. I will say only that I was trained in the latter school and find the treatment satisfactory. In any case, your physician is the best judge of what will work for your child.

Certain convulsions require further investigation by the physician: those that occur *without* fever and febrile convulsions that occur too often, too severely, or with too low a fever. In these situations, blood tests, electroencephalograms, X rays, or even trials on various medications may be necessary.

GENERAL HINTS: THE CARE OF SICK CHILDREN

Medicine

If the doctor has prescribed medication, follow the instructions exactly. If the prescription says "as necessary," use the medication *only* as necessary. Otherwise, finish the prescribed amount. If the instructions are not clear, find out exactly how much medicine to give, how often, and for how long.

Some medicines can be safely kept on hand and used from time to time: nose drops and decongestants for colds, antihistamines for allergies, cough medicines,[1] stomach settlers, thick mixtures to stop diarrhea, and laxatives. If your child has a recurrent problem, find out from your physician which mixture or brand of medicine he wants you to use.

How about the child who is difficult when it's medicine time? ("Doctor, I just can't get medicine into him. Please give him a shot.") Sam Levenson tells a story about the mom and dad who stand on their heads trying to get the

---

1. There are different cough medicines to stop cough, loosen mucus, ease wheeze, sedate, and so on. Do you know which you want to do? If not, find out. More on this in Appendix 2.

little monster to take two baby aspirin. No luck. When they throw the pills on the floor and walk out of the room, beaten, the child picks up the pills and eats them.

Children will do anything once they have learned that it is their *only* alternative. They must meet a blank wall in every other direction. Sometimes the medicine has to be forced a few times, or even refed after it has been vomited. (A new dose, that is.) Sometimes that blank wall has to take the form of physical force. But children learn quickly and are usually anxious to earn their parents' approval, so don't despair. You perform, and they will.

Here is a technique I have found useful for giving medicine, administering nose drops, and clearing out the nose with an aspirator or rubber-bulb syringe (see Figure 5). Wear an apron, and have a towel handy. Put the child on a kitchen counter where the height is right; immobilize his right arm against your body; firmly hold his left arm with your left forearm, leaving your left hand free to control his head. Prepare the medicine beforehand so that you can give it easily with your free right hand. If you're a southpaw, obviously you'll have to reverse everything.

A good trick for giving liquid medicines to infants and toddlers is to use a medicine dropper. They are available in different sizes, and some pharmaceutical companies provide them with the medication. (Most medicine droppers these days are plastic and therefore harmless, but be careful because there may still be some glass ones around.) Even if medicine is prescribed in teaspoonful amounts, it can be measured out by the teaspoon first and then sucked up into the dropper and squirted into the side of the infant's mouth.

Plastic injection syringes are also useful because they squirt so well. Most physicians use plastic disposable syringes; ask yours to let you have one (well rinsed, needle

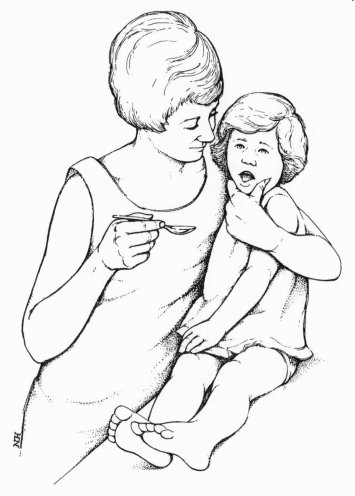

Figure 5. Administering medicine

off, of course). Squirt the medicine into the inside of the child's cheek. If the medicine tastes good, you'll end up with the child wanting to lick the tip of the syringe. You should then find it easy to switch to a teaspoon.

Finally, there is the problem of proper and improper dosage. Physicians and pharmacists are trained to prescribe and dispense medication accurately. Their instructions to the patient's mother should be precise. If an instruction seems wrong, or if you don't understand it completely, you should question it. The pharmacist has the right, even the obligation, to question the physician if anything seems unusual about the instructions for dispensing medicine. Anyone who is taking care of children should assume that same obligation. If there is *any* question, ask. It's better to risk asking a foolish question than making an unfortunate mistake.

Fever

Remember that fever is not necessarily bad. A little (101 to 102° F.) can easily be tolerated without aspirin and may actually help fight infection. Dress the child lightly, keep the room cool, and he'll be comfortable.

On the other hand, higher temperatures can be uncomfortable, dehydrating, and in some instances dangerous. Most doctors believe they should be treated with aspirin.[1]

Very few children are unable to tolerate aspirin. I find little reason to use anything else. Even a two-month-old infant can take half a baby aspirin without difficulty if it is crushed up in a little water. Baby aspirin tablets have now been standardized to one and a fourth grains (seventy-five milligrams). Any reference in this book to baby or children's aspirin implies this strength.

A safe dose of aspirin is approximately one grain (sixty

1. There is no liquid form of aspirin. Aspirin is acetylsalicylic acid. Liquid forms are aspirin substitutes with different chemical formulas. I believe they are less effective.

milligrams) per year of life, to be taken every four hours. Use the following table as a guide:

Approximate Age	Dose of Baby Aspirin
1 year	1 tablet (1¼ grains)
2½ years	2 tablets (2½ grains)
4 years	3 tablets (3¾ grains)
5–6 years	4 tablets (5 grains)
7–8 years	6 tablets (7½ grains), or 1½ adult aspirin
10 years and over	2 adult aspirin

Four baby aspirin tablets are the equivalent of one adult aspirin tablet. Five or six years may be a good age to switch to the adult form. Children should learn that medicine need not be pleasant-tasting.

Most children are not given aspirin around the clock; that is, six times in twenty-four hours. Even if they are, the dosage is still safe. The common symptom of aspirin overdosage in the younger child is rapid, deep breathing; in the older child, ringing in the ears. I have never seen these symptoms occur at the dosages I have recommended here.

Food

Many of our parents lived by the slogan "Feed a cold and starve a fever." It never made sense to me. The primary requirement for sick children is *adequate fluid intake,* and it doesn't matter how they get it. Clear liquids are usually a good start (including carbonated beverages or ice pops, all they want). When they get hungrier, milk, soups, gelatin, custard, and cereal are the logical next step. Contrary to popular belief, milk does *not* increase mucus in most children. However, it does in some.

Most childhood illnesses are short-lived; the child will not starve on a liquid diet. A good gauge of adequate fluid intake is adequate urination. Most children urinate several times a day, whether they are sick or well. If the rate decreases during illness, they need more fluids than you've been giving them.

Clothes

Keep the child cool when he has fever. As his temperature starts going up, you should start peeling off his clothes and covers. When his temperature reaches 103° F. or 104° F., the child should be naked. (Discretion is recommended in infants and toddlers not yet toilet-trained.) A light cover, such as a sheet, will keep the child comfortable until his fever goes down.

Activity

Most small children regulate their own activity very well. You cannot keep them up when they are sleepy, and they will cover seven to eight miles a day within the confines of their beds when they feel up to it. I have very few rules about keeping the sick child in or out of bed, in or out of doors.

Clinical studies have been made of traditional bed-rest diseases like nephritis, rheumatic fever, and hepatitis; bed rest per se has been pretty well discredited. I don't mean to suggest that rest is not important. But rest can often be made much more acceptable to a child who is allowed to be up and about.

Just as there is nothing magic about the bed, so, too, there does not appear to be anything magic about the house. Children can be brought out to the doctor's office just as they are brought out to the hospital when necessary; this does not seem to hurt them or make their condition worse.

I see no reason why children, even with fever, need to be kept in when the temperature outside approximates the temperature inside. As a matter of fact, when it is very warm, the child with moderate fever is often better off on a porch or outside under a tree than he is in a hot bedroom. The sick child needs, and wants, to be kept quiet. The best place for him is the place where this can be most easily accomplished. Similarly, air conditioners and fans can make the environment and the patient more comfortable in hot weather, and I see no reason why they should not be used.

Regulating the activity of older children who are recovering from longer and more serious illnesses (such as viral pneumonia, mononucleosis, hepatitis, and rheumatic fever) is more of a problem. In the negotiations that are sure to occur, the parent is well advised to think out the battle beforehand. Because total rest is impossible, compromises should be made carefully. The child will comply much more readily if leeway is *planned* and if limits *seem to be* negotiable.

In all things, common sense is the hallmark of good treatment. One of the first lessons the medical student learns is that nine out of ten patients will get well regardless of what the doctor does to them. (These figures are even better in pediatrics.) Let's try to maintain the statistics.

ACCIDENTAL POISONING AND DRUGS

All too frequently, an older infant, toddler, or young child gets hold of and swallows harmful drugs or chemical compounds. Parents need to know what action to take when this happens. They also need to know about unexpected reactions to drugs and improper drug dosage.

Types of Drug Reactions

Five types of drug reactions occur that need to be defined in a general way for orientation purposes.

1. *Desirable and expected.* The drug does the job expected of it when administered in the proper dosage. For example, penicillin cures streptococcal infections.

2. *Allergy.* After repeated exposure to a drug, a patient may develop common allergic reactions to it, breaking out in hives or a rash, and possibly experiencing swollen joints.

3. *Intolerance.* The patient who cannot tolerate a drug experiences side effects so unpleasant that he is unable to continue taking the medication. My daughter is intolerant of erythromycin; it gives her a bellyache. We have tried to fool her by giving her different brands in different forms, but her stomach knows. (Note that this is intolerance, not allergy.) If for any reason it were important for my daughter to have erythromycin we could probably give her other medications to relieve or even prevent the bellyache.

4. *Idiosyncrasy.* This reaction is similar to intolerance, but it is usually more severe and frequently occurs at the time the drug is first administered. A peculiarity in the makeup of the child causes the reaction. Thus, some children with bleeding problems cannot take aspirin because

it makes them bleed too readily or for too long a period.

5. *Poisoning*. Two situations are involved here: the taking of drugs or chemicals without parental knowledge, and overdosage, or as a result of unclear instructions or faulty interpretation of them.

Half of all children over a year of age who die, die of accidents or poisoning. Of all chilren who poison themselves, the peak age of incidence is about two years. And in cases of poisoning in toddlers, the most common substance is baby aspirin.

This kind of poisoning can occur even with the most careful mothers. For example, the baby aspirin is kept in the locked medicine cabinet. Just as the mother is giving the toddler his proper dose of aspirin, the five-year-old comes in with a cut on his head and blood streaming down his face! Mama goes to the five-year-old, and the toddler starts eating aspirin.

In addition to aspirin, toddlers harm themselves, sometimes fatally, with substances they find all over the house: cleansers (under the sink in the kitchen and bathroom), furniture polish (in the lower cabinets), mothballs (in the bottoms of closets), birth-control pills and tranquilizers (in the night table), plant and animal poisons (in the garage and basement), caustics (lye and ammonia), and fuels (gasoline and kerosene).

Obviously, parents must direct every effort toward prevention (specific instructions appear at the end of this chapter). I tell my patients' parents that their houses should be "poisonproof," whether they are there or not. We all know that no mother has her toddler in sight all the time, and that's when the poisoning invariably occurs.

Diagnosis of Poisoning

Most cases of poisoning are diagnosed when a parent finds an open pillbox or medicine bottle. Telltale evidence will be on the floor, on the toddler's clothing, or in his mouth. Occasionally, the container will not be obvious. Some of the wilier bandits will even throw it away—they know they've done something wrong, and so they destroy the evidence. In such cases, the diagnosis is made when the child develops the symptoms of sudden critical illness:

1. *State of consciousness.* Every pediatrician fears the next toddler who will swallow sleeping pills. It happens time after time. The only observable symptoms may be difficulty in walking and, sometime later, sleepiness. But frequently the child goes into deep unrousable coma. When this occurs, without any other sign, symptom, or laboratory test indicating illness, the odds are that the toddler has taken some pills. Doctors may never find the source, because some parents are so overcome with guilt that they won't admit to leaving the pills within easy reach.

2. *Respiratory distress.* I recently saw a four-month-old infant who was suspected of having pneumonia. He had had fever for four days and was already on antibiotics that were not doing a thing for him. When I saw him, his breathing was deep, hard, and fast (sixty to eighty times per minute). The examination was otherwise unremarkable. After he had been sent off for blood tests and X rays, my nurse asked me whether I thought a dose of three baby aspirin every four hours for four days wasn't too much for a four-month-old infant! It took us two days to wash the aspirin out of him with intravenous fluids.

3. *Fluid intake and output.* The sudden onset of very severe vomiting and diarrhea when associated with a change

in consciousness could mean that the child had taken a drug or eaten the leaves, flowers, or buds of some plant. The clues here are the suddenness and violence of the retching and the very obvious fact that the child is critically ill. In this situation, you are pretty helpless. The child needs medication that will have to be given by injection. Call the doctor!

Many drugs used commonly and uncommonly can affect the child's kidneys, which virtually shut down. In such a situation, sooner or later the mother notices the sparsity of urine being voided. (This is an example of how a drug idiosyncrasy can produce a disturbance of fluid balance.)

Treatment of Poisoning

This section is presented in checklist form for purposes of easy reference in an emergency. Follow the steps exactly, and in the order given.

1. *Make the child vomit.* There are only two exceptions here: *petroleum products* (gasoline, kerosene, benzene, oily substances, and cleaning fluids such as carbon tetrachloride) and *caustics* (lye, Drano, and ammonia). Everything else should be vomited. The best way to make the child vomit is to give him one tablespoon of syrup of ipecac. Repeat in thirty minutes if the child hasn't vomited. (Please note: *syrup* of ipecac, not ipecac *fluid extract,* a much stronger substance, which should never be used. It is much too powerful, and you will overdose the child.)

If you don't have syrup of ipecac on hand (you should), make the child drink a warm soapy solution or stick your finger down his throat, holding him upside down so that he doesn't choke.

2. *Identify the poison.* If it's a chemical, the container

should list the ingredients. If it's a pillbox or medicine bottle, call the pharmacist and find out the name of the medicine, its strength, and how much was dispensed. Then try to figure out how much was legitimately taken and how much is left or was spilled. If you can't reach your pharmacist, continue with this checklist.

3. *Call for help.* Try your doctor first. Tell the receptionist or answering service it's an emergency, a case of accidental poisoning. If your doctor or one of his colleagues is not readily available, ask her if she knows the number of your local Poison Control Center. If she doesn't, ask her the number of your local hospital or emergency room. The local directory-assistance operator will also have these numbers among her list of emergency numbers.

4. *Follow instructions.* You may be sent to a pharmacy to get syrup of ipecac, to a local doctor's office, or to an emergency room. Take the container of chemicals, the pillbox, or the medicine bottle with you. The pills can often be identified by comparison with a pill chart, the medicine by smell.

5. *Nonvomitable poisons.* If the antidote is listed on the label, use it. If not, give the child bland fluids such as milk, beaten raw egg, or (if available) a suspension of charcoal. Commercial poison-control kits have ipecac and charcoal ready for use in prescribed doses, and are available from your pharmacist without prescription. They're good to have on hand, especially if your child has swiped medicine before.

Prevention of Poisoning

The best "treatment" for poisoning, of course, is prevention. Certainly a preparedness-action program is in order for all children, and especially for the child who has already poisoned himself once. Repeaters are common. Here are some things you should do when your child first begins to move about the house independently.

1. Get some syrup of ipecac and charcoal suspension. Put it in a convenient location, and be sure that all adults, older children, and babysitters know where it is.

2. Copy the "Treatment of Poisoning" section from this chapter and tape it to the inside of the medicine cabinet door. Keep your poison-control kit (syrup of ipecac and charcoal) here too. Purchase your baby aspirin in small bottles with safety caps, and make sure all medicines are properly labeled.

3. From time to time, check the contents of all cabinets that are accessible to the baby who can crawl or walk. Make sure aerosol cans, detergents, furniture polish, and other cleaning supplies that are harmful if sprayed or swallowed are out of reach.

4. Fathers should check the garage and basement to make sure that they are poisonproof. And they should know about accidental poisoning that can occur when toddlers help their fathers work around the house. This is important.

Just as you have learned to drive defensively, learn to think defensively about accidental poisoning. When the children are grown, you can burn the instructions along with the mortgage.

2

The Ears, Nose, and Throat: Upper Respiratory Infection

A wise old pediatrician once said that most children have had a hundred upper respiratory infections by the time they are ten years old. I believe he was right. Certainly most sick children that I see in my office have runny noses, sore throats, coughs and/or earaches.

The fact is that most of them don't need to come in to the doctor's office. The treatment of these conditions hasn't really changed much in the last twenty-five years. It's true that great advances have been made in treating the *complications* of upper respiratory infection, but most children with colds have illnesses that really are not complicated and would get better with remedies their grandparents used. Why then does the major part of every pediatrician's sick call consist of a bunch of kids with runny noses? Are parents so insecure about the health of their children? Are they being overprotective? Are they really so concerned about the complications of the common cold?

All of these factors probably apply. But the common

denominator is parents' lack of experience in dealing with common childhood illnesses, along with the desire to secure the best and most modern treatment. And parents, not really knowing what the natural courses of these illnesses are, often cannot decide when they're simple and when they are likely to become complicated.

So let's take a look at upper respiratory infection in children: how it affects the ears, nose, throat, and sinuses; why runny noses are an integral part of growing up; how, more often than not, they can be treated safely at home without professional help. In order to do this, some basic understanding of the mechanism of immunity and its development is necessary. It is also essential to understand the structure and function of the organs involved and the ways in which they respond to infection. Then, it is hoped, the treatment will follow logically.

IMMUNITY: ARE THESE INFECTIONS REALLY NECESSARY?

Children are born with very little immunity. They have some antibodies (chemical particles in the blood specifically keyed to combat specific infections), which they have received from their mothers. Most of these antibodies disappear during the first year of life.

Infants do, however, have plenty of raw materials with which they can make their own antibodies. In order to make specific antibodies for specific infections, they need a pattern or model. This is provided by the infection itself. Just as a locksmith needs the lock in order to make a key that fits, so the body needs the infection in order to produce the right pattern for the antibody that will fit it and thus fight it.

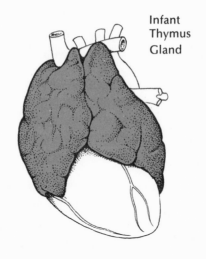

Infant
Thymus
Gland

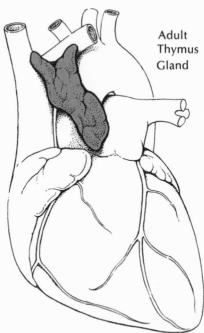

Adult
Thymus
Gland

Figure 6. Relative size of the infant and adult thymus glands

These raw materials are formed mostly in the thymus gland, which is located at the junction of the neck and chest, and in lymphoid tissue, which is distributed all over the body. The function of the thymus gland has only recently been made clear, and some interesting facts are worth mentioning here. The gland is enormous in the newborn in comparison with its relative insignificance in the adult (see Figure 6). Many doctors think that as immunity is acquired and antibodies are formed, the raw material is used up and the gland shrinks proportionately. It may be that the gland simply gets smaller as its work load decreases, but the speculation is interesting.

Such theories are attractive because they fit the patterns that pediatricians see in their patients. The relatively protected infant suffers comparatively little upper respiratory disease. In the early childhood years, when he becomes more social, his infection rate increases and peaks in the three-to-seven year age group. By the time he is eight or nine years old, he's likely to be absent from school very little and the worst is over.

THE ANATOMY OF UPPER RESPIRATORY DISEASE

The Nose

In addition to being the organ for the sense of smell, the nose functions as an air-treatment facility. Filtration is accomplished by large hairs at the entrance to each nostril, and microscopic ones (cilia) in the mucous membranes farther back. These cilia, by means of wavelike movements, can move foreign material forward, where it is discarded via sneezing and nose-blowing.

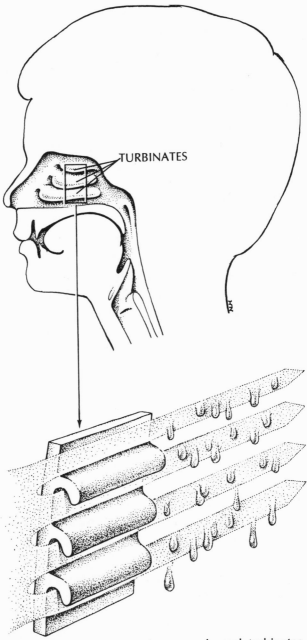

Figure 7. Air stream passing around nasal turbinates

The most ingenious accomplishment of the nose is the air-humidification process. Each nasal chamber has three curled-down shelves (turbinates) that project from the side wall, increasing the surface area. These turbinates are covered with a blanket of mucus-secreting cells that keeps them wet. Thus the air, passing across wet surfaces picks up moisture on its way down into the lungs (see Figure 7). This moisture is needed in the exchange of oxygen and carbon dioxide, and 95 percent saturation of the inspired air is achieved by the time it gets into the outermost areas of the lung.

Considering the constant intake into the lungs of low-humidity air (especially in centrally heated homes in the wintertime) and the exhaust of high-humidity air (blow on a cold window, and see for yourself) from the lungs, a tremendous amount of water is required. This explains the constant plea from doctors for more adequate humidification in the home. Not only does it soothe mucous membranes and make breathing easier, but it helps prevent dehydration in sick children.

The Sinuses

The paranasal sinuses are spaces or cavities within the bones adjacent to the nasal passages. They too are lined by mucous membranes and are connected with the nose by small openings. Their function is to help maintain a relatively constant air temperature in the nasal passages. I am sure that they become minimally involved when the upper respiratory tract in general is infected, but contrary to popular opinion, sinusitis hardly plays a *major* role in childhood upper respiratory infection. Occasionally, specific sinusitis causes more severe symptoms of fever, pain, and purulent (lots of pus) discharge. It then warrants professional help.

The Ear

The ear, the organ of hearing and equilibrium, is a complicated structure. The passages and chambers that are accessible to the outside world are most susceptible to infection.

The external canal, which extends from the outside ear to the eardrum, is long, narrow, and tortuous. The eardrum completely seals off the outside from the middle-ear chamber. But to allow proper vibration of the eardrum, this chamber must contain air, which comes from the nose via

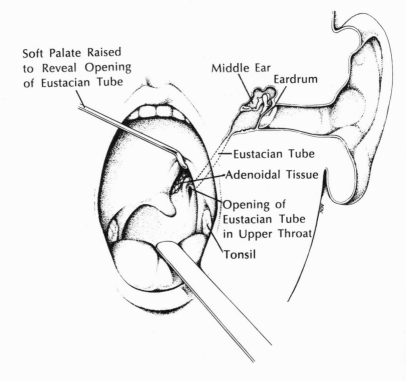

Figure 8. The ear and related structures

the eustachian tube (see Figure 8). The eustachian tube opening is very close to the lymphoid tissue—tonsils and adenoids—that make up the junction of the nose and mouth. When this tissue swells, it may seal off the opening of the eustachian tube, preventing air from getting into the middle ear. This is why people get earaches in association with upper respiratory infections; it is also the source of the problems people experience if they fly when they have colds. They have trouble equalizing air pressures on each side of the eardrum.

The Throat

The adenoids and tonsils are the sentries and arsenals in the fight against upper respiratory infection. The adenoids, which guard the nasal passage, can cause trouble by swelling and obstructing the flow of air to the middle ear, as previously mentioned. In addition, a child with swollen adenoids becomes a mouth breather and snores at night.

The tonsils guard the mouth and trap much of the infection that enters the throat. It is known that the tonsils played a role in modifying the intensity and severity of poliomyelitis, the disease that ran rampant during the thirties and forties. And it is known that childhood tuberculosis is likely to show itself first in glandular infection in the neck, before it causes major problems in the lung. The portal of entry is the tonsil.

This, then, is the anatomy. It will help you to understand how the problems occur and why we treat these problems in various ways.

SPECIFIC UPPER RESPIRATORY PROBLEMS

The Common Cold

It is not my intention in this section to describe all the clinical features of the common cold. Television commercials probably provide you with as good a reference source as any. I do want to show you how to decide when a cold is more than a cold and how to ward off complications when possible.

First, it is important to know that the infecting agent in a common cold is always a virus. (It may be one of many kinds.) Viral infections do *not* respond to antibiotics. They are, nevertheless, bona fide infections and may therefore produce fever. Common cold fevers in children are usually low-grade (100° to 102° F.), although they may be higher in infants and toddlers. But even though there is an infection and it produces fever, this by itself is no reason to prescribe an antibiotic. This is proven repeatedly in clinical practice. For example, antibiotics will not bring down the fever that accompanies measles or chicken pox (both viral infections). And remember, antibiotics are not always harmless.

Once it is understood that a cold produces swelling of the mucous membrane of the entire upper respiratory tract and that this swelling is accompanied by an increased outpouring of mucus, then all other symptoms can be explained logically.

As the mucous membranes increase their outpouring of mucus, the nose runs both forward and backward. Forward secretions run down on the upper lip and are obvious; backward secretions run down the throat and irritate. This produces a hacking cough and throat tickle. Swollen nasal passages make breathing difficult and sometimes even close the tear ducts. If tears cannot leave the eyes via their usual route into the nose, they will spill out over the lower eyelids and run down the cheeks. Because of the obstructed nose, breathing occurs through the mouth and throat instead of the nose, which causes scratchy throat. The adenoids swell and intermittently close the eustachian tubes, causing popping and plugging of the ears.

The cold progresses. Clear, runny mucus frequently becomes superficially contaminated with bacteria and turns pussy and thick. Usually a normal part of the cold progression, this heralds the drying-up phase just prior to the end of the cold. It is therefore not a sign of a complication and does not indicate the necessity for a trip to the doctor's office. It is perfectly reasonable for you to adopt a wait-and-see attitude, at least for a few more days.

How long do most colds last? It seems to me that the younger the patient, the less the immunity, and, therefore, the longer-lasting the cold. Most adults throw a cold off in a few days. School-age children's symptoms last slightly longer. The four- to seven-year-olds are coughing, sneezing, and blowing for a week at least; and infants' and toddlers' colds frequently don't dry up for two weeks. Within these guidelines, plus or minus a few days, it seems to me that as long as the child doesn't seem to be getting worse, watchful waiting remains your best course of action.

There are many treatments and medications that will help relieve cold symptoms. Aspirin reduces fever, relieves aches and pains, and promotes a feeling of well-being. (Note that it is important to take a child's temperature from time to time during the illness to see what his base line is.) When the mucus is thin, clear, and runny, decongestants taken by mouth may diminish the secretions. They are also useful in preventing ear infections in children who have a past history of this problem. Swollen nasal mucous membranes may also be helped by nose drops, which may also help prevent sinus infections in children who are susceptible to them. Nose drops are most useful in the later stages of the cold when the secretions become thicker, yellower, and more puslike.

The complications of a cold that should be treated by a physician are the persistence, prolongation, or intensification of symptoms in any one direction. Thus, when low-grade fever (101° to 102° F.) becomes high-grade fever (103° to 104° F.), or when occasional popping and plugging of the ear become intense, up-all-night ear pain, you should call the doctor. Coughs generally last slightly longer than colds, but when the intermittent, occasional, dry hacking becomes a persistent, deep chest cough with lots of mucus, the upper respiratory infection may have changed into a lower respiratory one. Alternate swelling of the eyes is sometimes an indication of deep sinus infection, which requires more intense treatment.

Finally, and most importantly, you should keep in mind the signs of serious illness. If the child's behavior changes radically, if there is any evidence of a lessening of normally alert behavior (especially if accompanied by the sudden reappearance of high fever and/or a stiff neck), this should be brought to the attention of your physician at once.

As for over-the-counter medicines, although their formulas may have similarities, there are subtle differences. Your physician is the best judge of which ones are right for your child. His choice will depend upon your child's makeup, his particular strengths and weaknesses, his specific reactions to various types of drugs, and so forth.

The next time you see your doctor, ask him which of these medicines he would like you to have on hand. He will be happy to help you. Your pharmacist may also have some good suggestions. He is well trained in pharmacology, and, in addition, has the practical knowledge of which patent medicines work best for his customers. He won't steer you wrong. In addition, the appendix lists a compendium of useful drugs and medications you may find helpful.

Remember, colds are colds. You can handle most of them yourself, at home, without calling your physician. Complications cannot be prevented by giving antibiotics but respond well to appropriate treatment when it becomes necessary. By and large, you will lose very little by waiting and allowing the cold to resolve itself instead of anticipating complications. So lay in your supply of tissues and go to work. And don't forget rest and increased fluids by mouth. They are always indicated.

The Nose

Two problems occur in the nose that are virtually unique to pediatrics.

FOREIGN BODIES. Beads, parts of plastic toys, screws, nuts and bolts, pussy willow buds, pieces of cotton swabs, marbles, and pills are all objects I have retrieved from children's noses at one time or another. If you are lucky, the child will tell you about it; and if the location is right, you may be able to get it easily. Don't try, however, unless you're sure that you can see it and that you are dealing with a cooperative youngster.

If you do try to remove it, here are some hints. Get comfortable, and make the child comfortable. Have plenty of light. Use a round-tipped tweezer, and try to grab the object. If it is smooth this may not be possible, but you may be able to work it out by getting behind it and pulling or pushing. A little blood with the procedure shouldn't upset you. If you don't get the object out quickly (first or second try; three strikes and you're out), quit! If you push it farther in or lose sight of it, or if there's enough bleeding to obstruct your view, call your doctor. It may be tougher than you think.

But if you succeed, and I hope you do, remember that where there is one foreign body, there may be two. So after it's out, take another look. And don't forget the other nostril.

Sometimes you find out about the foreign body days, weeks, or even months later. I once retrieved two pussy willow buds that had been in a nostril for two and a half months. The clue here, almost always, is a persistent, pussy nasal discharge from *only one nostril*. Any unilateral nasal discharge that lasts longer than a week should be brought to your doctor's attention. Don't try to get the object out yourself. It's too far in; the membranes are swollen around it; the tissues are sore, tender, and bleed easily; and if the object is breakable, it will break during the procedure. Leave this one for the doctor.

NOSEBLEEDS. Nosebleeds are common in children. Almost all occur under circumstances like these: The child has a cold or a runny nose. It is wintertime, and the humidity in the house is too low. The mucus dries just inside the nostril, on the septum (the dividing wall between the nostrils), in an area particularly rich in superficial blood vessels. The dried mucus, sticking to the membrane, causes an irritation that itches. The child then picks, wipes, sneezes, blows, gets hit, or in some other way pulls the mucus free. A piece of membrane comes along, and a small

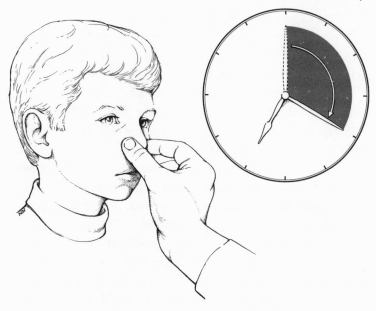

Figure 9. Stopping a nosebleed

vessel gets torn. The nose bleeds. More often than not this occurs at night, in sleep. And I've not yet heard of a case in which the amount of blood lost has been important. Usually it's just a few drops on the pillow.

My feeling about the treatment of nosebleeds is that simple pressure does the job nearly every time. Sit the child up, and pinch both his nostrils with your thumb and fore-finger. The pressure should be firm but not hard enough to hurt the child. Tell him to breathe through his mouth. The secret is to hold the nostrils pinched for twenty minutes, by the clock, without looking to see if the bleeding has stopped *during the entire twenty minutes* (see Figure 9). Every time you look to see if the bleeding has stopped, you disturb the clot, which may start the bleeding all over again. Clots frequently aren't firm for fifteen to twenty minutes.

This technique will stop most nosebleeds; the others will respond to a second twenty-minute period. Obviously, this treatment will not work for older people with arteriosclerosis or hypertension, but for children it works fine.

For the persistent nosebleeder, some other tricks are useful. Get the humidity up, especially in the child's room, and especially at night, with a vaporizer or humidifier. Put him on nose drops for a day or two in order to cut down on the mucus and shrink the blood vessels. If he's a known nose picker, especially in his sleep (and, strangely enough, many children are), put a drop of Vaseline on the septum of each nostril before he goes to bed. This will lubricate his finger (check the fingernail). Finally, if the blood usually comes from the same side, your physician may be able to find the bleeding vessel and cauterize it, ending the problem once and for all. If you take the child to the doctor with possible cauterization in mind, don't do it at the time of the nosebleed. There will be a clot there which the doctor won't want to disturb. Wait a few days; you may save yourself a trip. Finally, any nosebleed that cannot be stopped after an hour, any nosebleed that produces multiple clots leading you to estimate an ounce or more of blood lost, or any nosebleed that occurs in a child with a known bleeding problem should be brought to the attention of your physician.

The Ear

The worst common ear problems in children are related to respiratory infection occurring on either side of the eardrum. Let's consider these first.

MIDDLE-EAR INFECTIONS. Most middle-ear infections

in children are caused by lymphoid tissue swelling in the back of the throat and closing the eustachian tube. When the eustachian tube is closed, the air normally contained in the middle ear chamber is slowly but surely resorbed. Because additional air is not available, a relative vacuum is created. Normal pressure on the outer side pushes the eardrum inward slightly and produces pain. Since nature abhors a vacuum, serum from the membrane lining of the middle ear seeps into the chamber to fill up the partial vacuum.

The middle-ear chamber has access to bacteria, which can be found throughout the respiratory tract in any area that communicates with the outside world. This provides a perfect setup for infection. Bacteria are present and cannot be kept out of the middle ear. These bacteria have good nutrients in serum and are in a human incubator at ideal body temperature. They thrive and multiply. An outpouring of white blood cells, one of the body's natural defense mechanisms, helps to convert the serum to pus.

In the initial stages of serum and pus formation, the child is not likely to be in pain. The production of this fluid material eases the pressure differential, and the eardrum is no longer distorted. But as this pussy material multiplies, the pressure can actually be increased in the middle ear and the eardrum can bulge in an outward direction. This will cause pain again, and fever will be present or imminent.

If this process continues and the eustachian tube does not open, perforation of the eardrum can occur, with pus dripping out the external ear canal. There may be some blood or pus on the child's pillow in the morning. Interestingly enough, when the eardrum perforates, the reduction of pressure generally alleviates the pain. This appears to be nature's way of draining the pus from the infected area.

Many people are quite concerned about perforated eardrums because they have heard stories about their never healing and producing permanent impairment of hearing. Actually, this does occur, but only rarely and mostly in older children and adults with long histories of ear problems. Children with acute ear infections whose eardrums perforate usually heal their perforations very nicely in a few days.

But doctors know, as a result of preantibiotic experience, that although most ears will drain themselves and heal spontaneously, some will go on to complications. Additional infection, extension of the infection into the mastoid bone, and adhesions (scar tissue) in the middle ear can limit the vibrating motion of the eardrum and cause hearing loss. These complications are relatively rare if the child has adequate antibiotic treatment.

Although some ear sensations may occur with the common cold (plugging, intermittent ear popping, etc.), when bad pain, recurrence of fever, and the intensification of all symptoms toward one ear occur, this is indication enough of infection, and it's time to call the doctor. The potential consequences of infection of the ear are great enough, and the benefit of modern antibiotic treatment is important enough, to warrant professional care. Certainly the use of appropriate antibiotics and decongestants in middle-ear disease shortens the course of the disease considerably, gets the child back into school within twenty-four to forty-eight hours, and prevents most of the complications that were common in the past.

As I indicated previously, middle-ear infection seems

to be recurrent in certain children. Every pediatrician is repeatedly faced with questions from distraught parents concerning the frequency and intensity of these infections, and the possible effect on hearing in future years. There are probably a number of reasons why certain children have more middle-ear disease than others. One factor is the age of the child. Different parts of the body grow at different rates of speed at different times of life. Tonsil and adenoid tissue grows most rapidly when the child is four to eight years old. And this coincides precisely with the increased incidence of middle-ear disease.

This time can, however, vary according to the birth order of the child. Firstborn children follow the usual pattern of getting most of their respiratory disease around the fourth to eighth years. But in a family with many young children only a year or two apart, upper respiratory and middle-ear infections occur at a much younger age; infants and young toddlers getting as many infections as their older brothers and sisters. We can only surmise that such children are being exposed to greater amounts of infection and contract disease earlier.

It is certainly true that allergic children or children with positive family histories for allergy get into more upper respiratory and middle-ear trouble than other children. But there also seems to be a predisposition to middle-ear disease that is not necessarily related to allergy. The parents of children who repeatedly get middle-ear disease often report that they had similar problems when they were young. It is assumed that there is something about the anatomy of the eustachian tubes and the back of the throat that is inherited—perhaps a predisposition of the eustachian tube to closure and, therefore, an anatomic predisposition to middle-ear problems.

One of the responsibilities of the physician in dealing with the parents of these children is to provide constant reassurance and encouragement. The child will get better; the overwhelming majority of these children outgrow their previous predisposition to middle-ear infection; and they usually outgrow it without suffering any permanent harmful effects to their hearing or health. The treatment of these children is really a holding action and frequently depends upon how hard the parents are pushing the physician to make the child well. If you keep in mind the tendency of most children to outgrow this problem and, therefore, the reluctance of the physician to get too vigorous in management, you can evaluate treatment more knowledgeably.

The treatment of acute middle-ear infection should be three-pronged. Pain should be alleviated immediately. This is usually done with aspirin, sometimes with ear drops, and frequently with mild narcotics. An infectious process is taking place, and the judicious administration of antibiotics is appropriate. Your physician is in the best position to select the antibiotic. Proper antibiotic treatment will depend upon the age of the child, the condition of the ear, and sometimes the results of laboratory tests to identify the infecting agents. Because the inflammation will be eased by drainage, some sort of shrinking of the nasal mucous membrane should be undertaken, using nose drops or an appropriate systemic decongestant. Physicians usually continue this medication for a period of more than one week, most likely ten days to two weeks.

Intensive and prolonged treatment is necessary for the complete obliteration of the infection, so don't be surprised at the duration of the treatment. This is especially true twenty-four to forty-eight hours after the pain has become just a memory. I like to follow up on ear infections with a second examination to make sure that the infection has cleared properly. In many instances, additional medication or treatment is necessary.

Sometimes the best medical treatment does not seem to be able to clear an ear properly, and it becomes necessary to drain the middle ear surgically. This procedure is called a *myringotomy,* and it's the sort of operation that old-time practitioners used to perform on the kitchen table. Now it's usually done much more precisely and with much less trauma, both physical and emotional, under general anesthesia. Even though a hospital admission is required for this, it is usually of very brief duration (a day or so), and, in my opinion, well warranted.

A recent advance that seems to be effective in the management of recurrent middle-ear infection is the insertion of a small plastic tube through the eardrum. It is left there for a period of six to twelve months. The tube facilitates drainage at all times and never allows pressure or infection to build up within the middle ear. In my experience, this tube has worked well; I know of no reason why it should not be used. In most cases, sometime between the sixth and the twelfth month after insertion, the eardrum ejects the tube and closes up spontaneously. Recurrence of infection following this spontaneous closure is rare. (See "The Tonsil and Adenoid Problem," later on in this chapter.)

TEMPORARY HEARING LOSS. Hearing is frequently *temporarily* diminished in the early phase of upper respiratory infections or in the late phase of the common cold. This is caused by the presence of fluid in the middle ear and disappears spontaneously. (Consider the muffling of sound that occurs if you get water in your outer ear.) Such a hearing loss is usually short-lived and requires no treatment beyond that given for the middle-ear infection.

An interesting phenomenon does occasionally occur, however, which can seem to prolong the hearing loss unduly. In this sequence of events, a child develops a respiratory or an ear infection, fluid accumulates in the middle ear, and hearing is diminished. The fluid may persist for a period of four to ten days, and the child will become tired of trying to hear and failing. He just plain stops listening. With adequate treatment of the middle-ear infection and appropriate decongestion, the child's hearing should return quite nicely, but the child still may not be listening. The mother brings the child to the doctor: she thinks his cold has made him deaf. When the child is tested, either with the voice or with an audiometer, he seems to hear perfectly well. The mother's face gets very red, and she also gets angry with the child for having wasted time and money. I mention this only to reassure you that the phenomenon is an honest occurrence, readily explainable, and the visit is perfectly justifiable in terms of the reassurance that can be given to a distraught parent. After a while, the child realizes that he can hear again, and the "deafness" disappears.

A final word about tests of hearing. The so-called whispered-voice test is only a reasonable "guesstimate" of hearing function; it has severe limitations. The whisper test merely tests sounds in the voice, or middle frequencies. Perception of high-frequency sounds, which are the first to be lost in chronic and recurrent middle-ear disease, are not measured at all. I therefore advise the parents of children who have chronic and recurrent middle-ear infections to have them tested from time to time with a proper audiogram. In this way, hearing capabilities throughout the entire range of audible frequencies can be observed carefully during the period of frequent infection. And deficiencies can be diagnosed and treated.

SWIMMER'S EAR. External otitis (infection of the external ear canal) technically does not fall within the category of upper respiratory disease. But it belongs in a discussion of infections of the ear in general. The infection is contained within the skin of the external ear canal, up to and sometimes including the eardrum, but is not usually present on the other side of the eardrum in the middle ear. Usually occurring in summertime in northern climates (it can be a year-round problem in southern climates), it is known popularly as *swimmer's ear*. Most parents are uninformed or misinformed about this condition, which is extremely common.

According to an oft-repeated fallacy, swimmer's ear is contracted from dirty swimming pools. Attempts to culture bacteria from swimming pool water, from locker rooms, and from water fountains adjacent to swimming pools, have indicated no source of infection. Swimmer's ear is more likely a fungus infection of the ear canal, acquired from another child. Most children who have the opportunity to swim during the summer spend a tremendous amount of time in the water. The combination of ear canals that stay both warm and wet and the close contagious contact of all the other kids in the neighborhood probably encourages the persistence of this infection year after year.

One simple way to distinguish an external ear canal infection from a middle ear infection is to wiggle the ear. External ear canal infections are characterized by swollen skin along most of the path of the canal. When this skin is moved, or when attempts are made to move it, it hurts! On the other hand, middle-ear infections for the most part are confined to the area on the inside of the eardrum, and wiggling maneuvers of the external ear do not seem to bother them.

When infections of the external canal become troublesome, they are probably not only fungal in origin but secondarily infected with bacteria also. This accounts for the swelling of the canal, the extreme tenderness, the occasional fever, and the fact that these infections respond to treatment with antibiotics. If they were purely fungal, the antibiotics would not be effective. Furthermore, doctors see many children who have evidence of fungus infection of the ear but are not bothered by these infections and have no symptoms. Superficial infections may be picked up on routine physical examination, or may go undetected summer after summer. To the best of my knowledge, no harm is done.

The first step in the treatment of this troublesome situation is the prescribing of an antibiotic to clear up the secondary infection. This must, however, be followed by treatment of the fungus, which usually means eardrops. There are perfectly good antifungal ear drops that can diminish and sometimes even clear up these fungus infections completely during the swimming months. I have, however, been impressed by the number of recurrences of these infections as soon as the ear drops are stopped.

A better solution to the problem was found by the Yale swimming team some years back. They were troubled by these infections throughout the year. But they learned to control and even prevent them by using ear drops containing a solution that changed the pH (acidity/alkalinity) of the skin in the middle ear. I have found that it is easier to put ear drops in preventively once a day in those children who need them and then let the children swim all summer than to treat external ear infections intermittently throughout the warm months. Your doctor should be consulted about the prescription of these drops.

Here are a couple of practical points that may help you in both diagnosis and treatment. In the summertime, when a child complains that he has gotten some water in his ear and has not been able to get it out, be on your guard. He probably did get some water in his ear, but most likely he also has some fungus infection, ear wax, or possibly foreign bodies—all of which contribute to a feeling that he has an ear full of *something*. It all probably means swimmer's ear, and should be seen by your doctor. At this stage, it may not be secondarily infected and, therefore, can be cleaned out easily. Hopefully, the phase of the disease that is quite tender and painful can be avoided.

ADMINISTERING EAR DROPS. Trying to get medicine into the lowest reaches of the ear canal can be a difficult task. Have the child lie down, with the ear that is to be

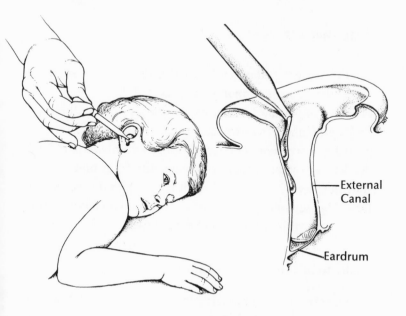

External Canal

Eardrum

Figure 10. Administering eardrops

treated facing up. The drops should be placed on the canal wall in small quantities and allowed to run down one side so that air can escape up the other side (see Figure 10). If air gets trapped below the drops, it will keep the solution from penetrating any further. If one or two drops are put directly into the ear, the ear canal may fill too quickly; there will probably be medication only in the upper quarter inch of the canal, the lower portion containing either foreign matter or trapped air. If this happens, the ear and ear canal should be manipulated in an attempt to squeeze the medicine down and allow the bubbles to come up. If the child's ear is quite tender to the touch, this can be difficult, but every attempt should be made to do it. Otherwise the medicine will not get to the place where it can do the most good.

SORE THROATS

In a recent pediatrics journal, a respected pediatrician made the statement that in the United States today, the only two important bacteriological causes of sore throat are diphtheria and streptococcus. A sweeping statement, but probably a true one. Diphtheria crops up only in small epidemics in isolated sections of the country from time to time; statistically it is not a problem in a well-immunized population. This section will deal with nonbacterial causes of sore throat and with streptococcal sore throat.

Nonbacterial Causes of Sore Throat

One of the commonest causes of sore throat in the northern climates during the wintertime is a factor I will refer to frequently in this section: low humidity in centrally heated homes. Usually at night, during sleep, the mucous membranes of the nose dry out and swell. Nasal stoppage causes mouth breathing, and low-humidity air irritates the mucous membranes in the throat. A child who sleeps in dry air often will awaken in the morning complaining of a sore throat. After breakfast his throat will feel better and will not seem to bother him through the remainder of the day. Simple as this is, it brings enough children into my office to warrant mentioning. Treatment is easy: set up a vaporizer or humidifier in a child's room (see Chapter 3), and the condition will be cured almost immediately.

Viral infections, of course, cause the overwhelming majority of sore throats. At this point, there are probably one hundred or more known viruses capable of causing upper respiratory infection and, therefore, sore throat. Only a few of these can be specifically diagnosed, but often, the presence of a virus is assumed when no specific disease is found on physical examination.

On the other hand, with many viral infections the child may have an inflamed and infected-looking throat, fever, pain, and swollen glands and is very sick. Here, one may have difficulty in trying to differentiate viral from bacterial (streptococcal) sore throat. Therefore, every child with a significant sore throat should have a throat culture made. Whether or not the throat is treated with antibiotics right away must depend upon the clinical judgment of the physician. He will certainly be justified in treating a child whom he considers to be quite ill while he waits for the results of the culture. He will be equally justified in withholding treatment from a child if he thinks a *viral* sore throat is likely. Because no bacteria are involved, the treatment of children with viral sore throat consists of gargling to relieve symptoms, aspirin for fever, and rest.

Infectious mononucleosis is one disease of viral origin

in which a severe sore throat is frequently the initial symptom. The throat may be quite inflamed-looking and swollen; it may be covered with whitish patches in the area of the tonsils. The child may have severely swollen glands in the neck and a high fever. The initial diagnosis is most frequently severe streptococcal sore throat. The patient is dutifully started on an appropriate antibiotic therapy, usually penicillin. The tip-off comes within twenty-four to forty-eight hours, when he doesn't get better. Penicillin is so specific and works so well against streptococcal sore throat that when it fails to perform properly, infectious mononucleosis must be considered a possibility. (Incidentally, a positive culture does not rule out mono, since 20 to 40 percent of kids with mono have strep, too, which has to be treated.)

Although it was previously thought that this disease was limited to older children and young adults, it is now cropping up more frequently in younger children. I've seen mononucleosis in a three-year-old. Perhaps we are recognizing infectious mononucleosis more frequently because a relatively simple diagnostic blood test that can be performed right in the office is now available. However, we don't do this test routinely since the overwhelming majority of sore throats are streptococcal infections.

It is not my purpose here to go into the diagnosis, treatment, complications, or prognosis of infectious mononucleosis. Most often its course is benign, it responds to rest and a "tincture of time," and no special medication is required. What you do need to know is that it usually begins with sore throat, does not respond to treatment with antibiotics, is frequently seen in older children (but may be seen in younger ones), and must be considered when the usual treatment of sore throat does not seem to succeed.

Streptococcal Sore Throat

Certainly one of the major advances in the care and treatment of children over the past fifty years has been the recognition of the importance of streptococcal sore throat and its usual complications. What *are* these complications? Why do physicians take such pains to recognize and treat streptococcal sore throat appropriately? Why is this disease recognized as the one upper respiratory infection that always demands adequate professional treatment?

It has been clearly shown that streptococcal infection precedes all cases of acute rheumatic fever and acute nephritis. Acute rheumatic fever is a generalized disease of the body that frequently affects the heart and thereby produces disease that may shorten life. Acute nephritis, although prognostically not so severe as acute rheumatic fever, nevertheless is capable of inflicting permanent damage on the kidneys, which also can shorten life. Furthermore, it has been clearly shown that the prompt diagnosis and treatment of streptococcal sore throat markedly diminishes the incidence of rheumatic fever and nephritis in children and teenagers. Therefore, every effort must be made at diagnosis and treatment to prevent the complications of both of these diseases.

The diagnostic problem is the difficulty in differentiating viral from streptococcal infections in some 80 percent of all cases of sore throat. That is to say, about 10 percent of all sore throats are sufficiently streptococcal in appearance for the physician to make the diagnosis with reasonable certainty. Similarly, about 10 percent of all sore throats are obviously viral. That leaves 80 percent of all sore throats in which the ability to make the diagnosis is strictly a toss-up.

Some physicians have better track records than others in attempting this diagnosis. But the probability of being right is not great unless an opinion is followed up with a laboratory-confirmed diagnosis. That is why doctors take throat cultures of most children who come in with the chief complaint of severe sore throat. Remember that the most horrendous-looking throat can be viral in origin, and the mildest-looking throat can be loaded with streptococcus germs.

The problem is even more complicated than that. Physicians recognize a condition known as the *streptococcal carrier state,* in which a child has a residual streptococcal organism in his throat. He has a positive throat culture time after time, but apparently does not have streptococcal disease. The bug hasn't really gone into the body, it just resides in the throat like a parasite, without harming or infecting it. The diagnosis of streptococcal carrier can be made with reasonable certainty also, but it requires at least two blood tests, with a period of ten days to three weeks in between them. If the patient has really had an infection, that's like closing the barn door after the horse has gotten out.

Obviously, this problem is complicated. Strep versus virus; infection versus carrier state. In a situation that can be so confusing even to doctors, how can a mother avoid being unduly worried when her children have sore throats and at the same time be sure that she is not neglecting a serious illness? How can she be helped to provide adequate medical care for these children without clobbering either the family pocketbook or her children's arm veins with needless and endless blood tests?

Any child who has a sore throat in conjunction with

fever and swollen glands should be seen by a doctor and have a throat culture made. The doctor is the one to decide whether the child should be started immediately on antibiotics or whether a wait-and-see attitude is appropriate. The results of the throat culture should be forthcoming within forty-eight hours.

A persistent but *mild* sore throat and chronically swollen glands unaccompanied by fever should also be brought to the doctor's attention. The throat culture can be taken by a nurse or an assistant in the doctor's office. (I think all offices should be set up in this way in order to allow more efficient use of the physician's time.) When the results are in, if the culture is negative, everyone can breathe easier; if the culture is positive, the physician will then examine the child. In this way unnecessary antibiotic treatment "just in case" will have been avoided.

There is one additional point that might be helpful to parents trying to determine whether or not a sore throat is streptococcal in origin: Is the sore throat accompanied by other upper respiratory symptoms? Ordinarily, if a child has many of the common features of an upper respiratory infection or cold (runny nose, runny eyes, slight cough, and nasal congestion), this disease is more likely to be a virus (rather than a streptococcus) infection. But if the child has a pure sore throat (with or without fever, but usually with swollen glands), the infection is more likely streptococcal.

Here are a few things you should remember about the *treatment* of streptococcal infection. Experience has shown that most cases of streptococcal sore throat will be cured (the streptococcus organism will be eradicated) with penicillin treatment in adequate dosages for ten full days.

Sounds easy. The difficulty is that the percentage of parents who give their children enough medicine for a long enough period of time (despite adequate instruction) is as low as 50 percent. When the symptoms subside in twenty-four to forty-eight hours, parents tend to become forgetful. And they worry about too much medication, penicillin allergy, etc. But they're worried about the wrong things. They may not know that there are still bugs around even though the patient feels better, and that inadequate medication will allow the streptococcal organisms to re-infect the throat at a later date. And they may not understand that inadequately treated infections that become chronic are frequently much more difficult to treat than acute ones the first time around. *Total dosage here is important!*

What about the other children in the household? Strep is contagious, isn't it? Yes, but not always. Much advice has been dispensed on this subject. There are those who would do nothing, and those who would give every exposed member of the family penicillin for ten full days. The middle-of-the-road path that I propose, and the one that seems most appropriate to the health of the children and the pocketbook of the parents, is to take throat cultures from all the children in the family and then treat only those whose cultures are positive. This system is not foolproof because it is possible for a child to contract the disease after the cultures have been obtained from a brother or sister whose culture will turn out to be positive. You can't really be sure there are no more streptococci hanging around unless all other children are recultured if a second case is found. And this could get burdensome. Nevertheless, it seems far more appropriate to take cultures than to treat everyone in the family. Otherwise an awful lot of penicillin would be prescribed needlessly. Doctors now have enough experience with streptococcal sore throat to know that it does not spread rampantly, although it certainly can, and does, infect other children within a family from time to time.

Another practice I have found useful is to reculture all children with streptococcal sore throat two to four days after they have finished their course of penicillin. I believe that the effort is worthwhile in order to pick up the 10 percent of children for whom ten days of treatment will not be enough. They may require other forms of therapy to eradicate the infection.

The children for whom ten days of penicillin is not adequate frequently respond to fourteen days or twenty-one days, and if this does not work, they may respond to changes in the form of penicillin administered by mouth, or even to long-acting injections of penicillin. One way or another, we manage to get them all.

THE TONSIL AND ADENOID PROBLEM

About fifty years ago, the practice of performing tonsillectomy and adenoidectomy on virtually every child whose parents could afford it was popular in parts of the United States. It was considered the best possible way to give children all of the advantages of medical science as the state of the art was known at the time. Over the years, however, the pendulum has swung back the other way, as it frequently does in such situations. When I took my training, the proper academic approach was conservative. Tonsillectomy and adenoidectomy were performed only when the most stringent criteria were satisfied and the child's condition was serious enough to warrant it.

Since then, I have looked at thousands of pairs of tonsils, thousands of aggregations of adenoids, and thousands of little children whose noses and throats contained this equipment. And through the years my ideas, too, have changed about the necessity of tonsillectomy and adenoidectomy.

There are many factors that have to be taken into consideration in making the judgment in the case of a particular child. But the complications of tonsillectomy and adenoidectomy have to be considered as well. The procedures are surgical, and every surgical procedure carries with it a certain risk of complication. They are accomplished under general anesthesia, and the inherent risk in anesthesia itself must also be considered. Further, it is possible that the tonsils and adenoids play a role in preventing other types of infection, possibly some infections still unknown to medical science.

It should also be clearly understood that tonsillectomy cures only recurrent tonsillitis, and adenoidectomy cures only problems related to enlarged adenoids, such as recurrent middle-ear infections. Neither of these procedures cures the common cold, runny noses, other viral infections, recurrent bronchitis, or other forms of upper and lower respiratory infection.

Therefore, the decision in favor of tonsillectomy and adenoidectomy is not a simple one and certainly should not be undertaken lightly. Although it may be helpful to get the opinion of an ear, nose, and throat specialist, the decision to perform surgery should be made by the child's doctor. The pediatrician or general practitioner is the one

who knows the child best, who sees the child most frequently, and who is therefore best able to evaluate all the
factors.

SWOLLEN GLANDS

More often than not, at some point in their lives, most
children will have glands that are swollen to a minimal or
moderate degree. These swellings may be located almost
anywhere about the head and neck. They are almost always
related to minimal infection. They come and go. They
may be swollen one day and not swollen the next. They
may persist for days or weeks in the presence of viral infection or local irritation such as bug bites, superficial
lacerations, and small infected areas. As long as the child
has some related symptoms such as a viral infection or
the obvious appearance of a minor skin infection, the
appearance of swollen glands is expected, understood, and
therefore not feared.

The only swollen glands that you need to be concerned
about are large and very firm and are associated with severe
tenderness, heat, and sometimes fever. These may persist
and stay enlarged for a relatively long period of time. These
glands (the large ones, the hard ones, the very tender
ones, or the ones associated with other significant general
signs and symptoms) should be brought to the attention of
your physician. But the smaller ones (the ones that come
and go, are not tender, are freely movable, multiple, and
widespread, and that cause the child no discomfort or dis-
ability) can be ignored until the next regular visit to the
doctor's office.

In summary, then, swollen glands in children do not usually signify serious illness as they may in adults. Unless they are very large (grape- to plum-size) or very tender and associated with fever, they do not require an urgent visit to your physician. They should be checked if they persist for a week or more.

3

Cough, Wheeze, and the Chest: Lower Respiratory Infection

COUGH

A cough is nothing more than a forceful propulsion of air outward from the lower respiratory tree—a mechanism, in fact, for getting rid of debris and foreign material. In order to do this, pressure must first build up within the chest. This happens when the airway is closed off. The chest then constricts, and the pressure is raised.

The voice box (larynx) is a structure that sits on top of the windpipe (trachea). It contains two vocal cords, semirigid structures stretched across the airway, attached in the midline on one side and able to open and close on the other. These cords act like curtain pulls, able to adjust the opening of the airway and thus modulate the voice as they vibrate in a stream of moving air (see Figure 11). For purposes of this discussion, think of them as able to close completely, actually closing off the airway to allow pressure to build up within the chest. When the cords are

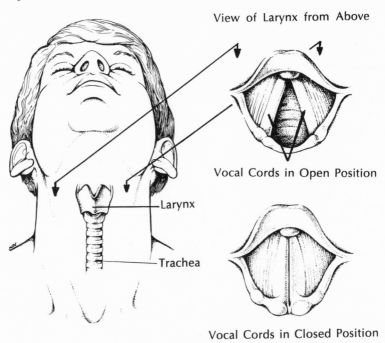

View of Larynx from Above

Vocal Cords in Open Position

Larynx

Trachea

Vocal Cords in Closed Position

Figure 11. The vocal cords

opened suddenly and completely with a good amount of pressure in the chest, a cough ensues. This sudden propulsion of air carries foreign material, debris, and mucus with it as it leaves the lower respiratory tract.

Coughs come in a variety of sizes and shapes. They may be loud or soft, dry and hacking, loose and juicy, occasional or frequent, croupy or brassy; and very frequently they are related to the position of the body if sinuses are draining. The loudness of coughs is only a measure of how much effort is being put into them. When coughs are dry and hacking, it usually means that something is irritating the respiratory tree. Sometimes the sensory nerves in the mucous membrane lining can't determine whether the irritation that triggers them is caused by the presence of foreign material or by the swelling and inflammation of the mucous membrane. Coughs that are loose and juicy indicate that mucus is being produced. The mucus that is ejected from the lower respiratory tract often flips over into the esophagus and gets swallowed. That is why many small infants with colds and other respiratory infections frequently have diarrhea that contains mucus. Mucoid material may also be seen in what they vomit.

POSTNASAL DRIP

The mechanism of this phenomenon operates exactly the way it sounds. Mucus from the nose drips down, irritating the throat and voice box area and causing a hacking, dry, nonproductive cough. Postnasal drip can occur at the tail end of a cold and last for days or even weeks. It can also occur in allergic children who have wet mucous membranes and whose noses seem to be dripping most of the time.

Here, too, body position is an important factor. Frequently, a child coughs only for the first hour or two after he goes to bed at night and again for the first hour or two after he gets up in the morning. This cough is usually the result of mucus accumulating in the sinus cavities, which drain when the body changes position and are so situated that some of them can drain when the child is lying down and others when he is standing up. Propping him up with a couple of pillows may be helpful. Try it.

Postnasal drip that is associated with colds will be helped by using a vaporizer or humidifier in the child's room at night to keep the mucus as thin as possible and therefore readily movable. If the mucus is thick and viscous (often it can be seen on the back wall of the throat), nose drops will shrink mucous membranes and help to liquefy the mucus. There are other decongestant medications that sometimes help to dry up the mucus when it is thin and runny (see Appendix 2). By and large, a chronic postnasal drip does not mean ear, nose, and throat problems for the rest of the child's life; rather it is another manifestation of the number of communicable upper respiratory infections that children have in the early years.

CROUP

The term *croup* applies to a wide category of childhood illness and probably describes many different infections. The common denominator in croup is a hacking cough, sometimes described as a seal-like bark, associated with difficulty in breathing because of obstruction to the airway. This obstruction takes place in the neck, precisely at the level of the voice box. The voice is usually hoarse.

"Midnight," or acute spasmodic, croup is a disease that occurs most often in the wintertime. Usually it is children in the two- to four-year age group who are affected. Usually the first sign of croup is the earliest sign of a viral upper respiratory infection: the child may have a slightly runny nose, more often toward the latter part of the day, and a change in voice similar to the change that occurs at the beginning of laryngitis. He does not, however, seem to be ill, usually eats a good dinner, and is put to bed without any difficulty. The characteristic cough typically begins around midnight, give or take an hour or two. The child has difficulty catching his breath between coughs, which scares him. (It has been said that difficulty with respiration is the most terrifying experience any human being can have.) The child's nose will probably be running both because of the infection and because he is crying, and he will be quite upset. He will have a low-grade fever (around 100° to 101° F.). At this point you must make a judgment as to how much trouble he is in. Generally speaking, if he can be settled down, and if his skin color is reasonably pink, or even a little red, there is no immediate cause for alarm.

One point should be stressed: when the child conveys his terror to the parent, if the parent, also frightened, conveys his sympathetic terror back to the child, the child will get worse. If there was ever a time to keep cool, this is it! Keeping calm is, in fact, an important part of the treatment and possibly the best thing you can do. On the other hand, if the child's condition seems worse after he has been awake for ten or fifteen minutes, if he spends most of his time trying to suck in air, if his color deepens and starts turning a little bluish, call your physician immediately.

Let me stress that the majority of cases of croup I see do *not* require my services and that the child would have done very well without them.

There are two important steps in the treatment of croup. One has already been mentioned—keep cool and do not transmit your anxiety to the youngster. Then: take the child into the bathroom, turn on all the hot-water faucets, close the door, sit down on the floor, and read him a story. Calmly. This makes most children comfortable enough so that they can very soon be put back to bed without any medication.

During this fifteen- or twenty-minute period, a hot or cold steam vaporizer should be set up in the child's room. If the child is very young, try to construct a tent out of sheets over the crib and direct the vaporizer into it, placing the machine far enough away, of course, so that the child can't get at it.

In the morning, he should be much improved, although he will have a residual cough. Sometimes the cough will seem to move farther down into his chest, which suggests a diagnosis of laryngotracheobronchitis, a type of croup that differs from the acute spasmodic croup. However, it is still *not* dangerous, is still usually viral in origin, and is still likely to get better by itself. In acute spasmodic or "midnight" croup, the child will usually get better quite rapidly over a two- or three-day period, and no other medication will be required. Laryngotracheobronchitis might take the better part of a week. See Appendix 2 for a discussion of cough medicines.

If the croup is unusually severe, if it is associated with moderately high fever (103° to 104° F.), if it persists into the following morning—and especially if still associated with fever—it may be of bacterial origin, which could be more dangerous. This croup does not get better dramatically, and, unlike the case of midnight croup, can be worse the second night than the first. It should be treated by your physician, who may give the child an antibiotic along with other medication to alleviate the symptoms as they occur.

I should mention that acute spasmodic croup, the simple kind, may recur beyond the two- to four-year age group. My first son had croup every winter of his life between the ages of three and nine. As a matter of fact, it finally got to the point where he would wake himself up, creep into our bed, and inform us that he had the "group" and would we please get out the vaporizer. He would go back to sleep cheerfully and awake in the morning ready for school. Obviously, he wasn't very sick. In later years, he didn't even bother with a vaporizer but would announce at the breakfast table that he had had the "group" the night before.

To summarize croup: It is an important disease. Usually croup is viral in origin, is accompanied by low-grade fever, is mild, will get better by itself, and needs no treatment beyond reassurance and high humidity. In its acute spasmodic or "midnight" form, croup is at its worst on the first night and gets better quickly thereafter, although a cough may persist for a few days.

The croup that is bacterial in origin is associated with higher fever and greater persistence of symptoms. The dangerous bacterial-origin croup is one in which respiratory distress is quite marked and the color of the child becomes dusky or bluish (in white children—in blacks, color won't help you).

On the evening that any croup first occurs, if the child can be settled down with reasonable ease in twenty or thirty minutes by means of reassurance and high humidity, he will probably spend a peaceful night and be much improved in the morning. If his symptoms worsen dramatically, your doctor should be called immediately. If they don't, but the fever and/or the symptoms persist in the morning, call the doctor then. If you are in doubt, no physician will mind being disturbed at any hour to help you evaluate the child's difficulty and treat it as necessary.

BRONCHITIS, BRONCHIOLITIS, BRONCHOPNEUMONIA, AND PNEUMONIA

Beneath the voice box, or larynx, is the main trunk of the respiratory tree (see Figure 12), the windpipe (trachea). This divides in the chest into left and right branches (main stem bronchi). These bronchi further subdivide into smaller bronchi. In the farthest reaches of the lung are the smallest branches (bronchioles), the final passageway through which

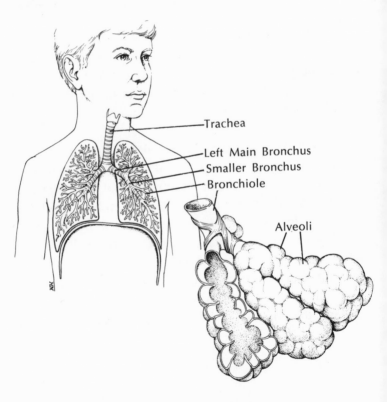

Figure 12. The respiratory tree

the air must pass before it gets out to the leaf (alveolus) of the lung. Tracheitis is inflammation of the trachea; bronchitis is inflammation of the bronchi; bronchiolitis is inflammation of the bronchioles; and pneumonia is inflammation of the alveoli. Bronchopneumonia is inflammation of both bronchi and alveoli. Thus, inflammation can have varying consequences depending on where it occurs and how much of each structure is involved.

Laryngitis, inflammation of the larynx or voice-box, commonly precedes croup or tracheitis. Its most prominent symptom is loss of voice, although sometimes pain is present. When due to an infection, it is almost always viral in origin. However, in children especially, yelling is frequently the cause. It should also be noted that allergy can produce, aggravate and prolong laryngitis: in these situations antihistamines are frequently curative.

Tracheitis is very similar to laryngitis and croup. It is usually viral in origin, accompanied by hoarseness and hacking dry cough, but not by fever. The condition will get better by itself. It responds to conservative measures and high humidity.

In *bronchitis,* the cough may begin dry, but soon becomes loose and juicy. The child may develop fever, and he looks sick. The cough produces a lot of mucus, is frequent and persistent, and lasts for days or weeks. Because of the large amount of secretions that may be involved, there is a tendency to secondary bacterial infection. Bronchitis usually responds to antibiotic treatment, though it is not always necessary. When your child has these symptoms and they persist, you should consult your physician. It isn't that children with bronchitis cannot recover by themselves: they can, and many children have bronchitis in these United States every year and get well without seeing a doctor. But if the physician feels that the secretions are bacterially infected, he will prescribe medication to shorten the course of the illness, make the child more comfortable, and avoid the effects of chronic bronchitis.

Bronchiolitis is a completely different disease. It is almost always viral in origin. It almost always occurs in infants and, very occasionally, small toddlers. And it is almost always associated with varying degrees of respiratory distress. The child breathes quite rapidly and makes a wheezing sound. The difficulty in respiration occurs both with breathing in and with breathing out. Note that this is different from spasmodic croup, in which the greatest difficulty is with breathing in, and from the wheezing of asthma, in which children have the greatest difficulty breathing out.

Respiratory distress in bronchiolitis can be a terrifying phenomenon. As shown in the cross-sectional diagram of large and small bronchi (see Figure 13), when the mucous

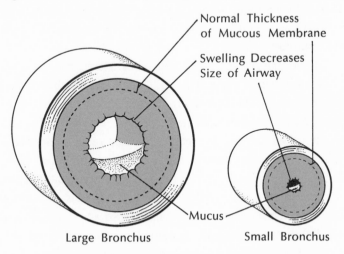

Figure 13. Large and small bronchi

membrane of the large bronchus swells, it cuts down the airway only very slightly. But when the mucous membrane of a small bronchus (bronchiole) swells, it may cut down the amount of space in which the air has to travel by 50 percent or more. If this process goes on in most of the lung tissue, there is precious little room left for the passage of air. This is why the child has trouble breathing. Since the disease is usually viral in origin, antibiotics will *not* help. Supportive measures and conservative care are the only treatments. Most children with moderate to severe bronchiolitis will be hospitalized, and indeed this is where they belong. In the hospital, their blood can be analyzed to find out whether they need oxygen and, if so, how much; their nutrition and fluid intake can be supported by intravenous feedings; and they can be watched much more carefully. The infant who wheezes, *has moderate to severe respiratory distress,* and intermittently coughs in a juicy or productive way should be seen by a physician early. He may be a candidate for the hospital.

Pneumonia is a disease that used to strike terror in our hearts, but really should not today. Its causes are well defined, its treatment is secure, and recovery from it is usually uncomplicated. There are essentially two varieties of pneumonia that you should know about in relation to children. Remember that pneumonia is an inflammation of the alveoli (the farthest reaches of the lung), and that bronchopneumonia is a mixed bag of bronchitis and pneumonia and usually is not a very severe disease.

Old-fashioned pneumococcal pneumonia is the disease that earned pneumonia the reputation it still has among laymen. In preantibiotic days, this disease lasted for weeks, during most of which the patient was very ill, with high fever, racking cough, and sometimes delirium. Its course built up in crescendo effect to a crisis from which the patient either recovered or died. This pneumonia is bacterial, usually caused by the pneumococcus organism, and usually accompanied by high fever, a hacking cough, and occasional chest pain. In the early stages of the disease, the physician may not be able to make the diagnosis because he may not hear anything with his stethoscope.

Many physicians do not order chest X rays very readily, and occasionally a day or two of watchful waiting is used to evaluate a child's condition. A chest X ray might reveal the cause of the fever and cough more quickly, but most often this is not necessary. When a child has a sudden high fever and persistent cough, the diagnosis to be considered most seriously is pneumonia, even though it may *not* be possible to hear the full-blown signs in the chest. Within a few days, if the disease is allowed to go untreated, the cough becomes productive of sputum and mucus. The sounds heard in the chest at this point would make the diagnosis obvious to a second-year medical student.

If the disease is caused by the pneumococcal organism, the treatment is penicillin or a comparable drug, and the child gets better quickly. The cough may persist for a week or so, but it becomes much less debilitating; the temperature goes down promptly, and the child generally feels better.

One of my professors once said that he had never seen the patient with pneumonia who didn't cough. By and large, I've found his statement to be true, although as I think back over all the children I've seen with pneumonia, it seems to me that I can recollect one or two in whom the cough was so minimal that it could be discounted. The important point to be made is that high fever and persistent cough that do not respond to simple home remedies within a day or two require examination by a physician. Complications are possible but highly unlikely. Professional treatment promptly restores the child to good health, and although the cough may persist for a couple of weeks, he will soon be able to resume his normal activities.

Bronchopneumonia is a much more baffling disease because of the variety of ways in which it may first appear. (I am lumping together a number of specific diseases under bronchopneumonia, since the appearance and treatment are generally similar.)

Bronchopneumonia, virus pneumonia, primary atypical pneumonia, "you've been walking around with pneumonia" —these are all expressions that describe an illness whose course runs something like this: One to three weeks after the onset of symptoms, a mother tells the physician that her child had a cold and had some fever for a day or two. He then seemed better and returned to normal activity except that he developed a cough which persisted. After a week or ten days, the cough became looser and juicier and even more persistent and the low-grade fever recurred. If the patient is a young child, he will have resumed his afternoon nap; if he is an older child, he will have taken to going to bed early. (All but undreamed-of in a child who is in good health.) The child does not appear very ill, but the physician can recognize the signs of pneumonia in one or more areas of his lung.

When I see these children in my office, they are not very sick. I treat them all with a four- to five-day course of an antibiotic that I know is useful in certain types of bronchopneumonia. Obviously, they don't all have this disease, but I cannot tell which do and which don't and so I elect to treat them all for a short course. If they don't have fever and feel generally well, they can go to school. They are just as capable of listening to the teacher as they are of watching television all day. But to prevent some of the complications that can occur with pneumonia of any kind, I ask that their activity be restricted to a minimum. The guideline instruction is that they are not to take *a single running step.* Rest is still a sound and reliable prescription, and the only way to rest the lung is to rest the entire body. So gym classes, bike riding, and paper routes are out. I expect to see these children in my office once a week until their chests are completely clear.

I tell the parents that the child with bronchopneumonia may continue to cough for one to four weeks, but that he will get better, and that his chest signs may also persist for that period of time. These children do *not* need additional and intensive courses of exotic antibiotics; they do *not* need single or multiple chest X rays repeated week after week; they do *not* need high-powered consultations with chest specialists. *They and their parents need to be forewarned that the disease takes time* and that *they will get better.* And the very act of forewarning provides the reassurance that most parents need in order to allow a physician to continue with the proper conservative treatment. Fortunately, the disease does not usually take as long as four weeks to clear, although it may.

Wheezing and Asthma

A sneeze, familiar enough to all parents, is a sneeze. Wheezing, on the other hand, confuses many parents. Medically, wheezing means noisy expiration (breathing out). Air has difficulty moving *out* of the chest. I think it bears repeating here that children with spasmodic or "midnight" croup have trouble breathing in, infants with bronchiolitis have trouble breathing in and out, and children who "wheeze" have trouble breathing out.

Wheezing is caused by spasm of the muscles in the walls of the bronchi and bronchioles. This spasm produces a reduction in the size of the airway, which, in turn, increases the velocity of the air traveling through the passages, makes more noise, and causes wheezing. In asthma and associated allergic disorders, there is an increased amount of mucus produced, usually thick and tenacious. This material produces a cough that may or may not be juicy and further impedes breathing by cutting down on the size of the air passages.

Any child with asthma (sometimes called *bronchial asthma*) needs to be treated by a physician. There are many aspects to the complicated diagnosis of asthma and allergies, many different ways that the symptoms and the disease can be treated, and many implications for long-term health that require competent medical care; wheezing children should be under the care of a physician. He will provide medications to be kept on hand, try to define and, if possible, eliminate the offending or allergic agents, and provide a careful follow-up during the worst phases of the disease in an attempt to prevent the long-term complications that may occur.

There are two other conditions, again peculiar to children, that should be mentioned in this context: *asthmatic bronchitis* (which is not to be confused with bronchial asthma) and foreign bodies breathed into the lungs or bronchial tubes.

Asthmatic Bronchitis

This is a disease that usually affects children in the two-to six-year range. Fever, a nonproductive cough, wheezing, and some difficulty in breathing are the usual symptoms. It is thought that this disease is basically an infection associated with an allergic reaction either to the infection or to the mucus that it produces. This combination sets up a spasm of certain bronchi and bronchioles and causes the child to wheeze. Most often accompanied by fever, asthmatic bronchitis usually lasts a few days and is readily treated with antibiotics and high humidity. It differs from asthma in that it occurs in younger children and is almost always associated with infection. The diagnosis of infection is made on the basis of fever and what the doctor hears through his stethoscope.

Although asthmatic bronchitis is found most commonly in allergic children, it does *not* mean that the child is going to develop chronic bronchial asthma. Even if your child develops asthmatic bronchitis a couple of times a year for a few years, the odds are still in his favor that he will not develop bronchial asthma as he gets older. He will probably manifest his allergic state in some other way (food allergy, drug allergy, poison ivy, eczema).

Foreign Bodies

Whenever a child chokes on a particle of food and then develops a sudden wheezing and cough that persists, it must be presumed that he has breathed some particle of food into his lungs. The foreign body may also be a small bead or part of a toy that the child has carried around in his mouth, as young children are prone to do, and that he then breathed in when he tripped or fell. It doesn't happen often, with food *or* objects, but the consequences of its going undetected could be serious. For this reason, any choking episode immediately followed by wheezing that won't quit, most especially in a child who has not previously suffered from asthmatic bronchitis or who is not known to have bronchial asthma, should be brought to the attention of your physician. A foreign body must be suspected.

TUBERCULOSIS AND ITS CONTROL

Tuberculosis is a complicated disease to diagnose because there are tuberculosis*like* organisms that may *act* like pulmonary tuberculosis, causing a positive reaction to tuberculin tests but producing no debilitation or pulmonary disease.

Urban children living under extremely crowded conditions are susceptible to tuberculosis, but the incidence of tuberculosis among suburban children today is very low. The statistics are rather amazing. Examining fifteen-year-olds in any city in the country at the turn of the century would have revealed that approximately 80 percent had come into contact with tuberculosis at some time in their past, had acquired minimal infection, and had produced resistance that kept them from contracting the disease we know as pulmonary tuberculosis. On the other hand, among high school graduating populations in suburban America today, the incidence of high school seniors who have been in contact with, acquired, and are protected from tuberculosis is 1 or 2 percent.

The reason for the improvement in such statistics, I believe, is the improvement in the techniques of early detection and, therefore, prevention. There is a simple, painless, and inexpensive skin test that can be administered easily to all children and that defines very clearly whether or not a child has come in contact with tuberculosis. Since we know the risk of infection to be highest in the first year following contact with tuberculosis, it makes sense to me to apply this test to every child in this country *every year*.

The administration of antituberculosis medication on a daily basis to all children who have recently had a positive skin test for tuberculosis has sharply diminished the incidence of serious disease in these children. The skin test is a far more sensitive screening device than the X ray, and there is no reason to expose children to radiation for screening purposes. X rays are important only when evidence of exposure to the disease, as produced by a positive skin test, is at hand. (See the immunization schedule in Appendix 1.)

For the sake of completeness, let me say that tuberculosis frequently hits children in the glands of the neck, rather than in the lungs. Therefore, the appearance of a relatively large (grape size or larger) gland, or series of glands, usually painless, but swollen, obvious, and persistent over a period of a couple of weeks, necessitates a visit to the physician for the purpose of checking out tuberculosis.

CHEST PAIN

I have to confess that I can find no good reason for the chest pain that occurs in most children I see with this symptom. Often the pain is real, but does not produce signs or symptoms that indicate its cause. And it certainly is not associated with disease that is of any consequence to these children. In any case, be assured that most chest pain in kids disappears without medical intervention.

There are some instances, however, in which chest pain is readily explainable. Perhaps the commonest one is the pain in the middle of the chest that is associated with the harsh, brassy cough of tracheitis or bronchitis. Since these diseases usually clear up by themselves, the pain disappears as promptly as the cough.

Another fairly common condition, *pleurodynia,* is a Coxsackie virus infection (see Chapter 6), which occurs in association with chest pain on one side or the other. This, too, clears up by itself and disappears with the virus. The pain, which can be quite severe, usually occurs when the patient takes deep breaths. Medication may be necessary to relieve the pain.

One final condition to be noted is *pneumothorax,* which may occur in older teenagers. In this condition, there is a weakness of the lining of the lung; physical effort, usually of no great magnitude, causes this defect to give way and burst. The lung collapses partially, causing chest pain, cough, and frequently shortness of breath. These symptoms come on quite suddenly. The appearance of the three of them in combination requires a prompt visit to the doctor. In some rare circumstances, pressure differentials build up within the chest that make breathing even more difficult. It has to be mentioned here that although these symptoms come on rapidly and may be quite incapacitating, many older teenagers and young adults do not seek help until their distress is overwhelming. Remember, the condition is serious enough to be brought to the attention of a physician *promptly.* Pneumothorax requires a chest X ray and, if a diagnosis is made, hospitalization for careful observation and possible treatment.

Let's put the statistics on pneumothorax into perspective. It is an uncommon occurrence in childhood and adolescence, and chances are you'll never hear of it again.

4

Bellyache: The Abdomen

Virtually all children have bellyaches. Bellyache may portend a surgical emergency; it can pose an elusive problem that may take months or even years to solve; or it may simply be the result of too much of the wrong food, too much excitement, or too much stress.

I'll deal first with serious causes of abdominal pain. These symptoms may indicate surgical emergencies and should prompt you to call your doctor sooner, rather than later.

Most bellyaches, of course, are not so worrisome. The main emphasis of this chapter will be on the more common, less serious causes of abdominal pain. In most instances, a parent who knows his child and is aware of the most likely causes of bellyache will be able to figure out what's going on.

BELLYACHES TO WORRY ABOUT: SURGICAL EMERGENCIES

Intestinal Obstruction

Normally, there is a continuous flow of food, liquid, or gases from the beginning of the gastrointestinal system (the mouth) down to the end (the anus). This dynamic action —sometimes rapid, sometimes slow—never stops. When it does, the child has intestinal obstruction and is in trouble.

Intestinal obstruction is always associated with vomiting and abdominal pain, and is frequently associated with abdominal distension (the blowing up of the belly to balloon-like proportions) and the cessation of bowel movements. But most important, it becomes obvious very quickly that the child is sick and that his condition is getting worse. When this combination of symptoms occurs, you should call your physician quickly. The specific diagnosis may not be obvious at that time and may require complicated tests. But that is a problem for your physician, not for you.

A distinction needs to be made here between intestinal obstruction and gastroenteritis. In gastroenteritis, most often the child will have diarrhea. The presence of diarrhea in fact *rules out* intestinal obstruction—the intestines are not obstructed if they are capable of producing diarrhea. The presence, then, of vomiting, abdominal pain, distension, and cessation of bowel movements suggests intestinal obstruction. In the section on gastroenteritis below, I will tell you how you can alleviate the symptoms of diarrhea. You can do nothing about the symptoms of intestinal obstruction except call your doctor.

Appendicitis

Appendicitis is probably the most common abdominal condition requiring surgery. Nevertheless, professors of surgery, who have seen thousands of cases, tell medical students that this may be the toughest diagnosis in the book.

Appendicitis is most often a disease of older childhood and most often occurs in boys. But it sometimes occurs in young children and in older adults, and it frequently occurs in young adults and in girls. Appendicitis is almost always accompanied by nausea and vomiting, but sometimes it is not. There is always pain and tenderness in the abdomen. But sometimes the pain is so minimal and the child so stoical that the pain hardly constitutes a major symptom. The location of the pain in appendicitis is usually in the right lower quadrant of the abdomen (see Figure 14). But sometimes the pain is most precisely located in the right upper quadrant or even in the left lower quadrant. The child usually has fever, although it is low grade (100° to 101° F.); but sometimes there is no fever at all.

From the foregoing, you can see that appendicitis can be very difficult to diagnose. The age of the child is a factor here. A teenager can give the examining physician a pretty good idea of his symptoms. But an uncomfortable, uncooperative, and unreasonable three- or four-year-old may be no help at all. There in fact appears to be an inverse ratio between the age of the child and the physician's ability to diagnose appendicitis prior to rupture or perforation. The younger the child, the more likely it is that the disease will progress to perforation before it is diagnosed. Even if the only symptom is pain, if it persists hour after hour, and it gets worse rather than better, your physician should be consulted.

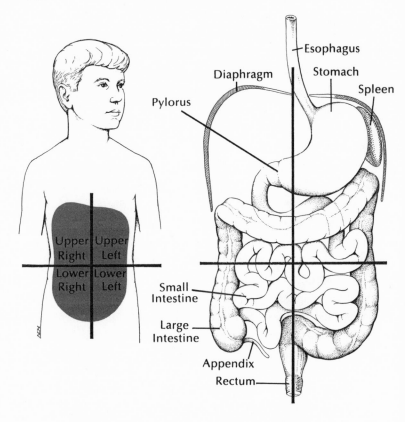

Figure 14. The abdomen and gastrointestinal tract

Any parent who thinks his child, regardless of age, may have appendicitis should call the doctor. The possibility will be suggested to you by the combination of abdominal pain, usually low and on the right side of the abdomen, and nausea and vomiting, in the *absence* of diarrhea. Watch for these symptoms in an older child, most especially in a boy. Your doctor may be able to make the diagnosis easily. On the other hand, he may have to make use of all his experience and textbook knowledge, as well as laboratory tests and a period of watchful waiting, before he can make a judgment. If in doubt, he may recommend surgery. This is the proper approach. There is a far greater risk in not operating on a child with a diseased appendix than there is in operating on one with a normal appendix.

Ruptured Spleen

Ruptured spleen is a condition that is less common than appendicitis, but it occurs frequently enough to warrant our discussion here.

Many children—especially older ones and especially boys—injure their abdomens in rough-and-tumble activity. If the injury occurs in the left upper quadrant (see Figure 14), and if the blow is particularly sharp, there is always a danger of rupture of the spleen. This injury is frequently seen as the result of accidents sustained in sledding and other wintertime sports, but it may occur in any season as the result of almost any vigorous activity.

In the typical case, there is an injury to the left upper quadrant, followed by the persistence of pain and tenderness in that area. The pain may be transmitted to the left shoulder or even down the left arm. One to several hours later, the child may become pale, sweaty, and clammy (symptoms of shock) and may experience some shortness of breath. This combination of symptoms should precipitate an urgent summons for help. Rupture of the spleen is an acute emergency and requires rapid surgery to remove the spleen and stop the bleeding. (Incidentally, as is the case with the appendix, people get along very well without the spleen.)

SIMPLE BELLYACHES: UPSET STOMACH AND THE BUG

The simplest kind of bellyache in children is the one that is associated with eating too much of the wrong food. Everyone knows that kids can eat peculiar things in fantastic quantities. Mark Twain spoke of "green apple" bellyaches. Today, these are more apt to be popcorn and candy bellyaches, ice-cream and cookie bellyaches, carnival or circus bellyaches. With stomach upsets like these, the history is usually clear-cut and readily provides you with the diagnosis. But some children will not admit to overindulgence in food. Sometimes you have to use your knowledge of the child and try to find out which foods have been available to him—or, as a last resort, examine the contents of what he vomits—to know what the offending agents were.

Upset stomachs are often cured by that tincture of time and judicious neglect. During the time that the child is suffering, he should eat no food, although clear liquids are okay. If the symptoms persist, your doctor may want to prescribe something to settle the child's stomach.

Gastroenteritis

Sometimes simple bellyaches turn out to be mild gastrointestinal infections (gastroenteritis), commonly called the bug or the *twenty-four-hour virus.*

Gastroenteritis can be defined as an inflammation of the gastric (stomach) and intestinal areas. The gastrointestinal tract is a long tube, with certain side attachments, that essentially begins at the mouth and ends at the anus. The mouth is connected to the stomach by the esophagus (see Figure 14). At the end of the stomach is the pylorus, a valve that acts as the dividing line between the upper and lower gastrointestinal tracts. In gastroenteritis, there is an inflammation of the gastrointestinal tract or some portion of it. This is almost always associated with increased activity of whichever section is involved and an attempt to reject its contents. By and large, the upper gastrointestinal tract rejects food by vomiting; the lower gastrointestinal tract by diarrhea.

Most gastroenteritis in children is caused by a virus, is brief, and is easily treatable at home. But gastroenteritis that is caused by bacteria (salmonella and shigella) usually has moderately severe symptoms and will require the help of your physician. You won't be able to tell the difference, so call him soon after the appearance of high fever or the continuation of vomiting and diarrhea beyond a twenty-four-hour period. The major hazard in gastroenteritis, especially in infants and toddlers, is the rapid onset of *dehydration,* which can be extremely serious (see below).

The treatment of gastroenteritis, then, is essentially the treatment of vomiting and diarrhea (described in the next two sections). Aspirin should not be given unless the fever is high (over 103° F.), because it may irritate the stomach. Rest is always indicated. Adequate liquids are important in all generalized infections, but even more so in gastroenteritis.

Vomiting

The frequency of vomiting in children seems to be related directly to age. Infants vomit or spit up for all sorts of reasons, including being overfed or underburped. Toddlers vomit when something bothers them, when they have upset stomachs, or as a symptom of other illnesses. Older children vomit when they have mild to moderate stomach upsets or gastrointestinal infections, or after eating too much. These types of vomiting are readily treatable at home. But when vomiting is persistent, when it seems to be getting worse instead of better, when it is associated with severe and progressive abdominal pain, call your doctor.

The diagnosis of vomiting can be difficult even for the physician. But parents do need to understand how this symptom may best be treated in children who are vomiting from any of a dozen unrelated and simple causes and who have no complications.

The first effort in the treatment should be directed against nausea. This can sometimes be accomplished by having the child suck on a hard candy or a lollipop for a half hour or so. He should not be allowed to chew it. Frequently, the sweet sensations to his tongue and nose pacify the urge to vomit. Follow the lollipop with the gradual feeding of chipped ice or flavored ices. Again, urge the child to suck and swallow slowly rather than to chew. If this is successful, begin an orderly progression of clear liquids in small amounts: water, flat (decarbonated) cola, ginger ale, Seven-Up, weak sweet tea, broth, or gelatin desserts in either solid or liquid form. The small-amounts-frequently concept should be followed rigidly. Try a teaspoonful every ten minutes. If the child keeps it down through a couple of doses, try a tablespoonful every twenty minutes. Finally, try one ounce every thirty minutes. To a small child who has just vomited, the sight of a full glass of liquid can be formidable.

This routine will stop simple vomiting in most children. If it doesn't, your physician should be consulted. He may feel that medication is necessary. It can be added to chipped ice and sipped slowly. Or, he may prescribe antivomiting suppositories. These, of course, cannot be retained in the rectum of a child who also has diarrhea.

A child who has recently vomited and who has graduated through the clear-liquid stage should not be put back on meat and potatoes too quickly. Rather, a slow progression of readily digestible foods that provide little roughage and few fats should be followed over the next two or three days. Cereals, soups, custards, puddings, soft-boiled eggs, and puréed foods are excellent. Once again, remember that severe vomiting, vomiting that does not respond to the simple routine, or vomiting that is associated with severe abdominal pain should be brought to the attention of your physician.

Diarrhea

Diarrhea is as common in infants and children as vomiting, if not more so. Its causes are varied. Infants sometimes have "intestinal hurry," which may be interpreted as diarrhea. Certainly many babies have diarrhea every time they teethe. And diarrhea frequently occurs with mild gastrointestinal disorders and simple gastroenteritis in infants and children of all ages.

When diarrhea is accompanied by vomiting, watch out! This is the setup for dehydration, which can be serious in infants and small children. When they are losing liquids by many routes—vomiting, diarrhea, fever, rapid breathing, and so forth—it doesn't take long for dehydration to set in (see below). Usually, however, simple diarrhea can be treated readily.

Remember this at the outset: No law says that stools must be formed. Infants and small children frequently have loose stools a few times a day, which may be perfectly normal for them until they get older. Diarrhea in an infant or small child who otherwise seems to be perfectly healthy is *not* a cause for great concern. Still, there are simple measures that may help alleviate the symptoms, and they should certainly be tried.

Food tolerance is the first thing to consider. For example, many infants cannot tolerate excessive amounts of fruit or fruit juice, and these foods should be restricted. For others, milk seems to be the offending agent and should be eliminated. Good supplemental nutrition will provide adequate minerals for strong bone and tooth building. Different foods offend different children, and when the diarrhea is persistent and troublesome, elimination diets may shed some light on the cause. This is frequently not necessary, however, if a child is doing well otherwise. "Doing well" can be defined as reasonable weight gain, growth, and disposition.

Teething, a common cause of diarrhea in infants, can be diagnosed merely by noting the association of the diarrhea with the eruption of teeth. The diarrhea will persist when the gums are swollen and stop when the teeth have broken through. No specific treatment is indicated.

The diarrhea of gastroenteritis may be slight or massive. There are instances of children having twenty to forty watery stools a day. These children invariably have trouble. If you think your child is losing more fluid than he is taking in, call your physician.

Early in my medical career, I encountered two schools of thought regarding the feeding of infants and children with diarrhea. One school said that all solids should be eliminated and the child kept on liquids until the diarrhea slowed up. The other school said that the judicious administration of certain solids seemed to make no difference and might actually help to firm up the stools. I lean toward the fluid-administration school because I believe that when a part of the body is sick, it should be rested. Since the work of the intestine is to digest food, the only way to rest the intestine is not to present it with food. It must be reemphasized, however, that although solid foods may be denied, liquids must be encouraged. It's easier to prevent dehydration than to cure it.

Many doctors feel that clear liquids (tea, ginger ale, broth, etc.) are the best liquids to use. Others advocate half-strength boiled skimmed milk. There are good reasons to use either or both. I think it's important to use the regimen that works best with the child.

Diarrhea in small children can always be eased with kaolin and pectin mixtures that help thicken stools and slow down bowel action. But most people don't use these mixtures in large enough doses. If you remember that these inert substances merely go in the top end and come out the bottom without ever actually being absorbed by the body, you'll be able to see your way to being more liberal with dosages. Kaolin-pectin mixtures often work satisfactorily, and may make more powerful medications unnecessary. (See Appendix 2)

Understand that a certain amount of diarrhea in an otherwise healthy infant or small child—if it does not seem to bother him and if he seems reasonably comfortable—may be tolerated and does not necessarily need to be treated. Often it is outgrown within a few months. The fact that a child *has* something does not always mean that you have to *do* anything about it. Many children tolerate mild deviations from what we consider to be normal behavior without any difficulty whatever.

Dehydration

Dehydration is a common complication of vomiting and diarrhea. Here again, the younger the child, the more likely he is to have significant dehydration along with vomiting and diarrhea. Infants and younger children require greater amounts of fluid per pound of body weight to survive: newborns require approximately two and a half ounces of fluid per pound of body weight in each twenty-four hours in order to maintain normal growth and metabolism; adults can survive nicely on half an ounce per pound. The infant's requirement, then, is in the magnitude of five times as much fluid per pound as the adult's. When an infant's fluid intake ceases (because of vomiting), and his output increases (because of diarrhea), his fluid balance becomes critical much more quickly.

The earliest sign that an infant or small child is becoming dehydrated is infrequent urination. A baby who always has a wet diaper, but who with vomiting and/or diarrhea starts having noticeably drier diapers, may be starting dehydration. A toddler or young child who usually urinates six to eight times a day, but who slows down to two or three times a day, may be dehydrating. Also note that the urine of children who are dehydrating often is darker than normal.

The second clue to the onset of dehydration is a change in the child's behavior (see Chapter 1). He becomes listless, is uninterested in his surroundings, and may have an increased desire to sleep. This latter symptom is the most confusing of all. Parents assume that if the child sleeps more than usual, it will help his recovery. Although this may be true of most other diseases, when an infant or small child who is on the verge of dehydrating sleeps, he is not being offered liquids and thus he is not drinking. Waking him frequently and offering him liquid is more important than letting him sleep.

More advanced signs, which should precipitate your urgent call for help, are sunken eyes, a sunken belly, and a doughlike quality of the skin. These signs indicate that dehydration has progressed to the moderately severe stage. This will almost always require hospitalization and intravenous fluids.

In summary, the end point in disorders of vomiting and diarrhea in infants and small children is dehydration. If either vomiting or diarrhea occurs in a child unaccompanied by dehydration, it can usually be treated successfully at home. When both occur simultaneously and are allowed to progress, dehydration will almost certainly result. The parent should, therefore, watch the child carefully, and keep urging him to drink. If one or both symptoms do not go away readily, call your doctor.

NAGGING, LONG-TERM BELLYACHES

One of the most common conditions that a pediatrician sees is chronic, intermittent abdominal pain. The diagnosis of this condition can be simple, or it can be one of the toughest in the book. I have seen children with chronic abdominal pain cured with one dose of a deworming medication. And I've seen other children go through exploratory surgery and still not get cured. Of course, the child whose symptoms are not eventually diagnosed is the one in a thousand. For most children, the nonpsychosomatic causes of chronic abdominal pain fall into one of three categories: constipation, pinworm infection, and (mostly in girls) urinary tract infections.

Constipation

When I was a young resident studying exotic and eso-teric disease, constipation did not exist as a cause of ab-dominal pain in children. It was a diagnosis made by old-school general practitioners who didn't evaluate chil-dren according to the newest "scientific" methods. Over the years, though, I've seen that proper bowel habits can do away with many chronic abdominal complaints.

I am not referring to the stool-retention syndrome characteristic of toddlers who are being toilet-trained. (The real problem there is with the training process and the amount of attention focused by young mothers on the bowel movements of their toddlers. A prompt deemphasis on training, eliminating all concern about bowel move-ments, invariably will enable a toddler to loosen up, and loosen his bowel movements as well.) I'm talking about the constipation that occurs in five- to 10-year-olds, and that causes chronic abdominal pain.

These children don't have the time—or, rather, won't *take* the time—to sit down, relax, and enjoy a good bowel movement. They may get up too late in the morning. They dawdle over breakfast. They fiddle around and almost miss the school bus. They are so eager to begin the activity of another new day that they can't waste time going to the bathroom before school. Unfortunately, school facilities and schedules are not conducive to unhurried evacuations, which means that such a child often does not have a bowel movement until immediately after school. But even then he is in a big rush. He may go to the bathroom when he gets home, but only to satisfy the parental requirement. He sits down, squeezes off a small bit of stool, wipes hurriedly (maybe), and then is out to play. He may have eliminated

25 to 50 percent of his rectal contents, but he certainly hasn't evacuated fully. Day by day, the residual stool builds up and, in addition, loses moisture (one of the major functions of the large bowel is to take water out of feces). The dehydrated stool may be very difficult, even painful, to move. So the child retains it.

You wonder, "Doesn't he have a desire to defecate after a while?" Remember that if you are in a situation in which you can't get to the john, you withhold the urge to defecate, and that after a while this urge diminishes. It happens with children, too. The nerve receptors in the wall of the intestine get tired of sending back the message that the bowel needs to be evacuated, and after a while they quit.

When a child's abdominal pain is due to constipation, the pain usually occurs around mealtime. He will frequently begin a meal, complain of pain, go up to his room and rest for a while, and then come down and finish the meal. When I see these children in my office, I always ask about bowel movements. The mother will quickly assure me that her child has one every day. When I ask about the nature of the bowel movement she often does not know, but the child will admit that they are small and hard. Cleaning these children out with laxatives, lubricants, or enemas will quickly alleviate their symptoms. But attention should be paid to establishing good bowel habits, which will keep the problem from recurring.

Which laxative? Which lubricant? An enema or a suppository? Different ones work best for different children at different times. When the problem is most acute, a glycerin suppository or one of the commercially prepared children's enemas will solve the problem. Prepared enemas are not dangerous, unlike old-fashioned large-volume enemas. The small amount of material that is squirted into the rectum cannot get very high up, near the area of the appendix. And there is no large volume of water to rob the rectum of precious salt. Still, if the problem is less acute, it probably should be attacked from above. I like to begin with lubricants because they are less likely to cause cramps. Some doctors advise giving mineral oil once every night in *any* amount necessary to make the child begin having comfortable bowel movements. He may actually leak mineral oil around his impacted stool before he begins to move it, but that is no reason to stop the mineral oil or even lessen the dose.

This treatment works well most of the time—if the child can be cajoled into taking mineral oil. It is important that the oil be administered only at bedtime, and to a cooperative child. If it is administered during the day, it may interfere with the absorption of fat-soluble vitamins. The child needs to be cooperative because mineral oil should never be forced down a youngster's throat. He may get it into his lungs, and oily substances in the lungs can be devastating. If this becomes a problem, a more pleasant-tasting laxative may have to be used. (See Appendix 2.)

If the abdominal pain is not severe, sometimes a combination of lubricants and mild laxatives will work more quickly. All physicians agree that the repeated use of stimulant laxatives is not desirable and may be habit-forming. They should therefore be used only on an intermittent basis. The best substitutes for enemas, suppositories, lubricants, and laxatives are the establishment of a good diet with plenty of fruits and vegetables and the provision in the child's daily schedule of enough time to contemplate and daydream while he has an adequate evacuation.

Pinworm Infections

The most sophisticated parent may recognize the fact that pinworm infections occur in children and yet refuse to believe that it can happen to his own child. Nevertheless, pinworm is probably the most common parasitic infection in North America. It is endemic to all sections of the country and to all socioeconomic levels. Although most common in four- to six-year-olds, I've seen pinworms cause definite abdominal pain in small toddlers and older teenagers. It has been said that if the dust from the classroom floors of most of our schools were collected and analyzed, the pinworm egg count would be fantastic.

To understand this disease, you need to know something about the life cycle of the pinworm (see Figure 15). This small, thin, threadlike worm, usually one fourth to one inch in length, lives in the large intestine. When the female worm is loaded with eggs, it migrates down the intestine, through the rectum, and out the anus, where it lays its eggs. It is a nocturnal creature; egg laying almost always occurs at night. The activity of the worm in and around the anus may cause intense itching. The worm then migrates back into the intestine and continues its life there. It may live for six to eight weeks. The life cycle is prolonged because the itching stimulates the child to scratch, and then, if he puts his fingers in his mouth, he carries eggs from his anus to his mouth, where the eggs are ingested. They pass down to the large intestine, where they are hatched—thus beginning the life cycle all over again. In addition, small children may pass the infection to each other because their fingers and their clothes are contaminated with the eggs. It is easy to see why nail biters and thumb suckers have the most difficult and recurrent infestations.

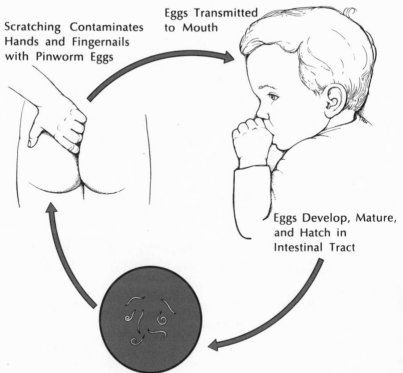

Scratching Contaminates Hands and Fingernails with Pinworm Eggs

Eggs Transmitted to Mouth

Eggs Develop, Mature, and Hatch in Intestinal Tract

Adult Worms Shown Here Actual Size Emerge from the Anus at Night and Lay Eggs on the Surrounding Skin.

Figure 15. The life cycle of the pinworm

The worm frequently resides at the top of the large intestine or the bottom of the small intestine, and, interestingly, this is the precise location of the appendix. Just as the appendix is capable of causing abdominal pain when it is inflamed, pinworms are capable of causing abdominal pain, presumably when they inflame the section of the bowel to which they become attached. In fact, they will in some cases get into the appendix and cause symptoms that precipitate surgery for acute appendicitis. An expensive way of treating pinworm, isn't it?

Here are the probabilities: Any child who complains of abdominal pain and is in the habit of scratching his fanny at night has pinworm until proven otherwise. Any child who has had pinworm and who complains of abdominal pain has pinworm until proven otherwise. Any child whose brother or sister has recurrent pinworm infestations and who then begins to complain of abdominal pain has pinworm until proven otherwise.

The simplest test is to look for the worms. Examine the child's anus very carefully, an hour or two after he has been in bed. If you see any, your doctor can recommend a vermifuge that will eliminate pinworms with one dose in the majority of cases. Call him in the morning. If careful inspection at night does not turn up any pinworms, you can perform simple tests under his direction that will enable him to make the diagnosis. Please note that the accuracy of the diagnosis increases with the number of tests taken. In my office, three tests are a minimum before the diagnosis of pinworm is ruled out.

There should be no stigma attached to a child who has pinworm. If he is not kept in a glass house, he is as capable as any other child of acquiring pinworm infestation. The important consideration is to diagnose the condition if it exists and to get rid of it.

It is generally accepted that once the diagnosis of pinworm infestation is made in a family, all the children should be treated. In many instances, infants less than a year old and older teenagers who have good hygienic habits may be excepted. On the other hand, if the infection seems to recur, not only all the children but also the parents and anyone else who lives in the house should be treated.

Despite all preventive measures, pinworms may occur time after time in one family. The source is usually the nail biter or thumb sucker, the child who continually has his hands in his mouth. In such a situation, treating the child routinely every six weeks (the normal life expectancy of the pinworm) should completely eradicate the infection —so that no eggs can be transferred from the upper to lower gastrointestinal tract during the time of treatment. It would also help to eradicate the pinworm egg population in the rugs and the upholstered furniture. Thorough and repeated vacuuming is the best way.

Urinary-tract Infection in Girls

In female children, urinary-tract infection is another common cause of abdominal pain. Why girls? Because of their anatomy. A diagram of the urinary tract shows that there is a reasonably long distance between the bladder and the outside world in males and a very short distance in females (see Figure 16). As a matter of fact, the distance between the bladder and the outside world in a female toddler or small child may be as short as a quarter to a half inch. Since the bladder is the reservoir of urine, this is an area in which bacteria that have gained entrance to the bladder may have the time to grow and multiply before being evacuated. And access to the bladder is very easy in the female.

There are other anatomical factors that may enhance the conditions under which urinary-tract infection occurs in girls. Sometimes girls have tight bladder outlets that do not allow them to evacuate completely. This causes a stagnation of urine, which, in turn, encourages the growth of bacteria within the bladder.

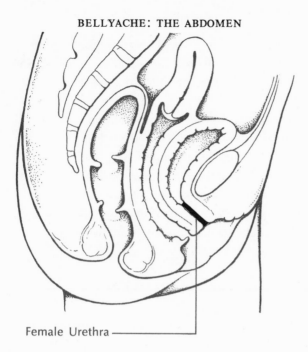

Female Urethra —

Male Urethra —

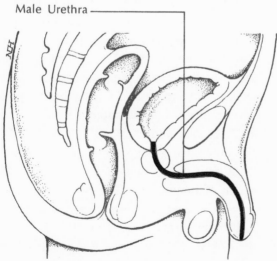

Figure 16. Relative size of the male and female urethras

The main point to be made here is that no investigation of chronic abdominal pain in a female child is complete without a careful look at the urinary tract and its functioning.

Many female children who complain of burning on urination and whose urine is found *not* to have infection are victims of bubble bath. Apparently, the detergents and chemicals in bubble bath are capable of irritating the mucous membrane linings of the vagina and urethra. These children's symptoms are alleviated by cutting out bubble baths. It's a small point, but worth remembering.

BELLYACHES THAT AREN'T BELLYACHES

Sometimes bellyache is the chief complaint, but the abdomen is not the source of the problem. Why this happens I don't know, although, like many pediatricians, I have a theory. It seems to me that an infant or small toddler's first lesson in anatomy from the parent often concerns the stomach. I think of simple expressions like 'What a fat tummy you have," "Is your tummy full?" or, when the child is distressed for any reason, "Does your tummy hurt?" And in toddlerhood, "You have to go to the potty and empty your tummy"; "Don't put toys in your mouth or you'll swallow them and they'll land in your tummy."

Maybe this emphasis explains why, when a child has a complaint about pain in any area of the body, he will frequently complain of tummyache. The best example of this is the toddler with a severe ear infection who is presented to the physician with a temperature of 103° F. and complains of a bellyache. The abdomen is normal; the ear is abscessed. Children with sore throats often complain of abdominal pain; children with incessant cough develop charley horses of their stomach muscles and complain of abdominal pain; certainly many children with headache complain of stomachache at the same time. This is common and should be remembered when a child who is obviously ill, usually with infection and fever, complains of abdominal pain and there is a noticeable absence of other symptoms related to the abdomen.

It is also true that children who are nervous, children who become acutely intimidated or scared, children who are apprehensive about social or school situations, children who get motion sickness (usually in an automobile), children who get too excited, and children who undergo too much physical activity may develop abdominal pain. Sometimes it's just a bid for maternal attention—what Dr. Rustin McIntosh calls a "mummyache," rather than a tummyache. This may have to do with nerve mechanisms in the intestine or changes in the distribution of blood supply between the intestine and the remainder of the body. Fortunately, these complaints about abdominal pain are short-lived and may be repetitive enough in similar situations for the parent to recognize them quickly.

Then, of course, there's the school-morning bellyache. Many children develop an abdominal pain in the morning before going to school that seems to get better very quickly after they have missed the school bus. Unfortunately, the abdominal pain of constipation occurs at mealtime, and thus the school-morning bellyache may be confused with the abdominal pain of constipation. Still, a parent can recognize that this pain does not occur on weekends, does not occur during vacations, and in the older child may occur in conjunction with certain homework assignments, examinations, or teachers. The treatment of this condition will depend on finding out what's going on at school.

BIG BELLIES: OBESITY MALNUTRITION

The most common form of malnutrition seen today in American children is obesity. Found predominantly in the "underdeprived" children of suburbia, obesity causes more serious disease than does the kind of malnutrition found in ghetto children. After all, if heart disease is one of the greatest killers of adults in this country; and if all the correlations now being made between heart disease and hypertension, cholesterol problems, and coronary artery disease, are accurate; and if these problems are in turn related to nutritional factors, then it must follow that obesity is a major cause of cardiac problems and therefore of mortality among adults.

I submit that obesity is a disease acquired in early infancy and childhood, a theory that is borne out by more studies every day. It is true that there are large gaps in our knowledge of the genetic, metabolic, and biochemical aspects of obesity. But within the confines of what we do know, much obesity is environmental. "Overnutrition" is taught by well-meaning parents who were similarly taught when they were growing up.

Keep in mind the fact that a person's lifetime eating habits are probably formed before the age of five! There are valid psychological reasons why this is so, and there is some evidence that overfeeding—even in infancy—produces physical changes in the body. These physical changes may persist throughout life and create a demand on the part of body organs for excessive nutrition.

Mothers should learn a lesson from the insurance companies—their statistics tell us that, so long as we're healthy, the skinnier we are, the longer we'll live. But it's very difficult to translate this fact into the technique of child rearing. After all, who wants a kid with his ribs sticking out? *But that skinny kid is healthier!* Fat does not protect a child from viral illness, the common cold, the flu bug, strep throat, pneumonia, or any of the other childhood infections he can be expected to contract as he grows and develops. The clean-plate club is a dangerous organization whose membership is encouraged by millions of parents in an effort to make their children eat.

There are distressed areas in this country in which one finds deficiency diseases. But when you consider the nation-wide problem, a far greater mortality will occur as a result of obesity in our children than as a result of deficiency disease.

5

Allergies

Allergy is an exaggerated response to a stimulus or foreign substance that may contact the body in several ways. The foreign substance or offending agent is called the *allergen*.

Let's look at different methods of allergic contact and a variety of familiar, straightforward allergic reactions.

COMMON ALLERGIES: DIFFERENT METHODS OF CONTACT

By Mouth

Children are frequently allergic to foods or to medicines taken by mouth. Shellfish, tomatoes, and strawberries are good examples of foods that can cause allergic reactions; penicillin and sulfa preparations are common causes of drug allergy.

Reactions vary from such local manifestations as lip

swelling, bellyache, vomiting, and diarrhea to a more generalized reaction involving hives, wheezing, and even shock or circulatory collapse. The reactions may be very specific (I'm allergic to crabmeat but not to shrimp), and they may be quantitative (I can eat a little crabmeat occasionally, but if I eat a lot of it, or eat it several days in a row, I get hives). Food and drug allergies are easiest to diagnose in older children and adults—you get reliable information as to which foods or drugs have been taken.

Through the Nose

Allergens may be inhaled. Pollenosis (hay and rose fever) and allergies to dust, grasses, weeds, and molds may produce sneezing, itchy and runny noses, swollen and tearful eyes, and even cough, wheeze, and chest congestion. Hay fever is so common that in some areas of the country weather forecasters routinely report pollen counts.

Through the Skin

Many common household and environmental substances can produce allergic reactions (skin rashes) just from contact; wool, cosmetics, and poison ivy, oak, and sumac are examples.

Other, more subtle, environmental allergies are produced by light and cold. My wife can tolerate temperate-climate sun, but the tropical sun gives her hives and a skin rash along with her sunburn. And I remember a man in the Air Force who had to be transferred from Germany to Africa because he started to wheeze whenever the temperature dropped to 30° F.

Injection

Offending allergens injected into the body can produce allergic reactions. Perhaps the best-known example of this is penicillin. Allergy to penicillin can manifest itself minutes after injection or weeks later. It may produce symptoms as slight as a mild itch at the site of the injection or as severe as hives all over the body, difficulty in breathing, even shock and circulatory collapse. Fortunately, severe reactions are rare in adults and even rarer in children.

Delayed reactions to penicillin may cause a condition known as *serum sickness* weeks or even months later. This is manifested by mild rash, fever, swelling of the legs and joints, and some degree of general debilitation. Sometimes the association with penicillin has been forgotten by then, obscuring the cause of the symptoms.

One final word about penicillin allergy: The allergists say that reaction to one type of penicillin probably means reaction to *all* types of penicillin. Newer penicillins, which are synthesized in the laboratory and not cultivated in molds, have different applications and uses and are considered by some to be completely different drugs. Don't believe it, say the allergists. Stay away from all types of penicillin if there is any history of allergic reaction to *any type*.

The foregoing are all common allergies, commonly talked about, and usually affecting older children and adults. As is the case with so many medical conditions, allergies in infants and small children may not have the same symptoms or offending agents.

CHILDHOOD ALLERGIES ARE DIFFERENT

In childhood, allergies differ according to age groups. The age groups do not have precise limits, and there is a tremendous variability in the severity of symptoms. Nevertheless, it can be stated generally that infants usually are allergic to what they eat, toddlers to what infects them, and older children to what they breathe. Obviously, this is a huge oversimplification of the problem. But it presents a good point of departure.

Food Allergies in Infants

Although infants are often allergic to things that contact their skin—like wool, baby lotion, powders and ointments, nylon and rubber pants—most of their allergies come from food. Since the food most commonly given to infants is cow's milk, cow's-milk allergy is the most common form of allergy in this age group.

I have never seen an infant who was allergic to his own mother's milk, nor have I heard of any such documented instance. (On the other hand, one of the things we are taught early in medicine is never to say "never.")

When adults are allergic to foods, their symptoms seem to be directly related to the offending allergen—for example, their lips may swell or hives may appear soon after eating a forbidden fruit.

An infant's symptoms are not so specific and are much less severe at first. They are, therefore, more difficult to diagnose. Infants who become allergic to cow's milk may have intermittent diarrhea (sometimes even constipation) and occasional spitting up, may be irritable, may seem slightly congested with mucus most of the time. Of course, all degrees of severity of these symptoms may be present. Thus, vomiting and diarrhea may be impressive, the "colic" may progress to "crying all the time," and "small amounts of mucus" may progress to wheezing and severe respiratory distress.

Although there is no specific and reliable test for cow's-milk allergy, some reasonably good ones are being investigated clinically and in laboratories. The diagnosis is usually made, especially if there is a positive family history for allergy, by trying the infant on a formula that is free of cow's milk. Substitute formulas are usually soybean preparations, protein complexes, or meat-based liquids. A child should not be considered allergic to cow's milk unless a trial on one of these other formulas produces dramatic improvement (although this improvement may take as long as three weeks to show up) *and* unless the child shows a definite return of symptoms when the cow's milk is tried again. (Obviously, medical judgment may dictate that the cow's milk formula not to be tried again if the symptoms it produced initially were severe.)

Many parents are apprehensive about raising their children on milk-free diets, but it is really much easier than it sounds. The infant usually takes to and tolerates a substitute formula quite well. The development of good bone and tooth structure does not seem to be compromised by the absence of cow's milk. Some infants may require supplemental calcium, but most seem to get enough of the minerals they need for sturdy bone and tooth development from other foods. And (as you will see) they are usually back on milk within a year.

Things get more complicated later in infancy when other foods are being introduced that may contain milk.

Initially, all dairy products—such as butter, cheese, and ice cream—should be avoided. Since many baked products and cereals have milk in them, they should be avoided too, at first. Fortunately, a combination of events occurs that usually eases parent and child out of a difficult situation. The infant doesn't want or require some of these more attractive milk-containing products until later in the first year. And since he seems to outgrow his milk allergy around the same time, a slow transition occurs in which he ingests and is able to tolerate milk and milk products. As a matter of fact, what usually happens is that the parents get more confident and start cheating a little. Thus, tastes of ice cream, nibbles of cheese, and "a little bit" of butter, "just for flavor," gets tried. Before long, the mother tells her doctor that the child takes all kinds of milk products without difficulty, and "couldn't we try a little milk?" The transition is smooth from then on.

It should be mentioned that quantity seems to be a factor here. That is, older infants seem to be able to tolerate small to moderate amounts of milk and milk products but frequently have a recurrence of their earlier symptoms if given too much too soon. This phenomenon is probably responsible for the old wives' tale about not giving an infant with "mucus congestion" too much milk.

Other foods most commonly associated with allergy in infants are wheat and eggs. Of these two, wheat is the more difficult to eliminate. It's relatively easy not to offer an infant egg, either pure or in combination form. But when he gets to the stage where finger foods are desirable, most of them will contain wheat. However, a sharp-eyed search through the fantastic variety of foods found in supermarkets will usually produce rice cookies and crackers and other wheatless bakery products on which an infant can teethe. Here again, allergy to these foods seems to be outgrown toward the end of the first year, making it possible for them to be introduced cautiously without too much difficulty.

Infection and Allergy in Toddlers

Some years ago, at the Babies Hospital in New York, I attended a seminar on recurrent upper respiratory infections. A visitor from the University of Saskatchewan in Canada told us about an interesting observation made at his medical center: many of the mothers of infants and toddlers with recurrent upper respiratory infections complained that they had experienced the same symptoms during their pregnancy. When investigation revealed the only factor common to these pregnancies to be the women's drinking large quantities of milk, chronic milk allergy in both the toddlers and their mothers was suspected. Sure enough, when these infants and toddlers were taken off milk, the number of their respiratory infections decreased dramatically.

Of course, it's not so clear-cut as it sounds. To my knowledge, a controlled study was never performed. But there has been a growing suspicion over the past ten or fifteen years that allergy plays a much larger role in childhood infection than has ever been realized.

Another clue to the relationship between allergy and infection in toddlerhood may be found in the type of respiratory infection that is acquired. Bronchiolitis in infants, croup in toddlers, and asthmatic bronchitis in preschoolers seem to occur in families that have positive histories of allergy. These same children develop other allergic manifestations later in life. For instance, there seems to be a correlation between the occurrence of these diseases and children who have eczema, which is generally recognized as a skin disease of allergic cause (see Chapter 8).

Older Children: Other Allergies

As with other types of diseases, the older the child gets the more his problems resemble those of his parents. Older children get hay fever, asthma, chronic eczema, poison ivy, oak, and sumac; and more of them become allergic to foods and medicine. But remember, only a small percentage of children with asthmatic bronchitis go on to develop full-blown bronchial asthma. And most children who develop bronchial asthma outgrow it.

This outgrowing phenomenon is interesting, and not always limited to children. For years I supplied a good friend of mine with his favorite antihistamine capsules to get him through the worst part of the hay fever season. One year autumn came and went before I realized I had not had my annual call and called him to ask what had happened. It seemed that during the previous season, my friend had found that he required so few capsules that he had not bothered with them during the current season. He guessed his allergy had just plain quit.

A RATIONAL APPROACH TO AN IRRATIONAL DISEASE

Any disease or condition that is incompletely understood and therefore confusing might be considered irrational. Actually, we learn more about allergy every day. If we put aside some of the dogma and rigid thinking that have characterized the treatment of allergy for many years and begin to consider some of the newer evidence and observations, a reasonable scheme for dealing with allergy in children emerges.

Are the Parents Allergic?

The tendency toward allergy is hereditary, and consideration of the family history is always important. After the first or second child in a family develops allergy, doctors and parents should look for allergic manifestations in subsequent children. But what about the first child? What about the family history of allergy in parents and grandparents, aunts, and uncles? It's easy to come up with a positive family history if there are relatives who have had common allergies like bronchial asthma, eczema, or penicillin allergy. But sometimes the family history is more obscure. Consider the pregnant women in Canada who had symptoms of upper respiratory infection during their pregnancies when they were drinking unusually large amounts of milk. Consider the people who go through life with chronic cough, with sinusitis, dry skin, skin disease of undetermined cause, or stuffy noses. Doctors are beginning to suspect that what many of these people actually have is manifestations of allergy in a mild form. Such factors should be considered in trying to determine a positive family history of allergies.

Babies of Allergic Parents-to-Be

Assuming an allergic family history, how should young parents-to-be approach the arrival of a new baby? There are those who would have them create an allergy-free room, start the infant on soybean-milk preparations, and otherwise prepare them for a highly regimented existence with their firstborn. These measures may not be necessary at all. In my opinion, this is a time for watchful waiting.

Breast-feeding should be encouraged, since allergy to breast milk is all but unknown. If breast feeding is not elected, some theorists think that formulas of condensed or evaporated milk and water sit better with the allergic infant than whole cow's-milk formulas. I won't argue, because I don't believe enough information is available to settle the issue one way or another. Both formulas are equally nourishing.

Certainly the newborn should be watched for the subtle signs of allergy that can develop in small babies. Eczema in florid patches of irritated skin occurs on the cheeks, *not* in the creases of the elbows and knees, as it does in older children. Mild to moderate intestinal disturbances also are common. New foods should be introduced one at a time. (If apples are fed for breakfast, peaches for lunch, and pears for supper, and on the following day a rash appears, you can't tell which food is the offender.) Another symptom you should be on the lookout for is chronic nasal and chest congestion in an infant who is not exposed to many people with colds. This allergic reaction is less common, but it certainly occurs.

Once it has been established or at least strongly suspected that an infant I'm treating has allergies, I recommend a diet free of milk, wheat, and eggs, since these are the foods most likely to cause allergies in infants. Mild eczema of the face usually requires little more than frequent washing with soap and water. (In my opinion the benefits of washing the face with soap and water outweigh the possible disadvantages of soap allergy.) I advise against the use of baby lotions, bath oil, and other scented skin prepaarations—they are more likely to produce allergy than to soothe the skin. This is as far as I think one ought to go in the treatment of the very young infant who shows signs of allergy, as long as these measures keep him comfortable enough to gain and thrive. If the allergies are more severe, your doctor can provide other means of relief.

ENVIRONMENTAL CONTROL

Even though infants are usually allergic to what they ingest rather than to what they inhale, you should start thinking about environmental control when you have an allergic child. There are four major aspects of the child's environment over which control should be exercised: humidity, air cleaners, wool, and pets.

Humidity

The first and possibly most important consideration is the provision of adequate humidity within the house. In an allergic family or a family in which there is an allergic child, year-round humidification should be provided. In homes heated by circulating hot air, excellent humidifiers can be installed on furnaces, which during cold weather will provide between 30 and 50 percent humidity. Adequate humidification will be enhanced by the installation of storm doors and windows. In houses that do not have hot-air systems, portable humidifiers can be provided for the bedroom area. If a good permanent site for the humidifier can be found, it is worth having a plumber install an automatic refill mechanism. You should also encourage members of your family to take showers rather than baths and, of course, use vaporizers and humidifiers when your children have respiratory illness. Another good method of providing humidity in a dry home is to unvent the drier so that it discharges into the house. Dry a load of sopping wet towels, and you will see how nicely the moisture appears on your cold windows. Fortunately, heating engineers say that humidity is relatively quickly and uniformly dispersed throughout the house.

Air Cleaners

Dust has been identified as one of the most common allergens. Use a vacuum cleaner, rather than a broom or carpet sweeper, to remove it. If your house has a circulating hot-air furnace or air conditioning, change the filters frequently.

In hot-air-heated homes, a device that works quite well as an air cleaner is the electronic precipitator. It is installed in the furnace to take the place of mechanical filters. In houses in which circulating air is not the method of heating or cooling, a portable precipitator can be rented or purchased and installed in the room of the child who suffers most from inhalant allergies.

The child's room needs other special considerations. It has been said that the perfect allergy-free room would resemble a jail cell. No clutter. Yet today, children's interests and activities are so varied that clutter is a way of life. Nevertheless, it can be controlled. Items of furniture with large surface areas collect dust. For example, venetian blinds should be avoided. Carpets, fuzzy stuffed animals, and bookshelves are also dust collectors. Children, like squirrels, have a tendency to collect things. Try to keep these collections on closed shelves, as much as possible.

Wool

Synthetic materials—which, unlike wool, are not allergenic—should be considered when selecting *any* floor covering or clothing for an allergic child. Infants with eczema should not play on wool-carpeted floors, wear wool sweaters, or be covered up with wool blankets.

Pets

Finally, a word has to be said about pets. This is sometimes a difficult, even heartless taboo to enforce, especially when allergies are discovered after pets have become members of the family. However, some pets seem worse than others. In my experience and in the experience of many pediatricians and allergists, the worst offenders are cats. There are *no* nonallergenic cats. It is almost possible to make the statement that any allergic child who lives with a cat will become allergic to that cat sooner or later. If you have an allergic child, don't get a cat. If you already have a cat, get rid of it if that is at all possible. And if you can't bring yourself to get rid of it, then try to keep the allergic child and your cat as far away from each other as possible.

Most dogs are allergenic, and dogs with long hair are as allergenic as cats. Some say that the poodle is an exception. I cannot see why, even if he has no dander and stays well clipped. But there are those who defend poodles on this basis, and I can't argue because I have no data that proves otherwise. The safest procedure, in my opinion, is to limit the pets in a house full of allergic children to goldfish and gerbils.

ALLERGY FALLACIES

Allergy fallacies have developed as fast as new allergies have been recognized. The consequences of believing some of these items of misinformation can be devastating; others are just unnecessarily bothersome.

Penicillin

Children are frequently suspected of having penicillin allergy on very tenuous evidence. Articles have appeared recently in medical journals about the misdiagnosing of patients as having penicillin allergy. It is easy to see how this can happen. Doctors see many children with diseases, accompanied by fever, in which a specific diagnosis cannot be made. Unfortunately, many of these children are placed on penicillin. Most common illnesses with fever in children are caused by viruses, and many of these viruses involve, as part of their symptoms, the appearance of a rash at some time during the illness. It is therefore easy to see how a child may become ill, be seen by the physician and started on penicillin, and a day or two later develop a rash. Frequently the doctor does not see the rash. He is consulted over the telephone, and makes the assumption that the child is allergic to penicillin. The child is taken off the penicillin, the rash goes away (as it does in most viral illness), and the child lives, possibly unnecessarily, with the stigma of being allergic to penicillin for many years, if not for life.

Sometimes it is possible subsequently to give the child a very minute dose of penicillin to see if the rash can be reproduced. This must, of course, never be undertaken without the specific direction of your physician, since theoretically it is fraught with danger. Actually, very few children have reactions to penicillin that are severe or life-threatening. That seems to be a more common occurrence in adults. If your physician chooses, penicillin allergy can be tested for by more scientific means under more controlled conditions. However, this is often thought to be unnecessary, since many new drugs have come along that can replace penicillin in most of its uses.

Skin Tests

Many children are diagnosed as having a dust allergy because they sneeze in dusty rooms, or possibly on the basis of skin tests. In an experiment once performed at Bellevue Hospital, children who were diagnosed as being allergic to dust were placed in environmentally controlled rooms in an allergy unit. The air was filtered, and the children seemed to do well. Porters were then sent out to these children's homes with vacuum cleaners to collect the dust from their homes and their rooms. This dust was brought back to the hospital and sprayed into the environment in which the children were living. Some of the children, as might be expected, reacted violently, proving the diagnosis. But a great number had absolutely no reaction to the very dust to which they were supposed to be allergic. Such is the state of the art, which is one reason allergic disease may be labeled "irrational."

Any pediatrician or allergist who is worth his salt will attest to the low degree of reliability of certain skin tests. What the professionals are really saying is that if an allergic patient is skin-tested and the results are found to be markedly positive to certain allergens, and if a vaccine is prepared and the child is desensitized to these allergens, and if the child gets demonstrably better, the skin test is reliable. But if the skin tests are negative, or if the desensitization program does not work, then the test must be considered unreliable.

Stinging Insects

A word needs to be said here about the bites of stinging insects. I am referring not to mosquitoes or fleas but to bees, wasps, hornets, yellow jackets, and all the other insects that have been incriminated in rapid, fatal reactions. A widespread and morbid fear exists about the possibility of a child's dying instantly following a sting—doubtless because of the rare but well-publicized instances of an adult's being fatally allergic to such a bite. At a conference I attended recently with other pediatricians and allergists, it was generally agreed that this is a phenomenon that occurs in adults, not children. We had collectively seen thousands of stinging insect bites in children and hundreds of allergic reactions to these bites, but only one person was able to recount an incident of a near-fatal reaction in a child.

So let's get the record straight. Allergy to a stinging-insect bite implies a reaction to that bite that is generalized, not local. Hives all over the body, shortness of breath, tightening up of the throat muscles, difficulty in swallowing, or any generalized symptoms should prompt you to call your doctor quickly. Local swelling, local itching, and local pain are simply immediate effects of the bite. Granted, they may sometimes be quite severe and may persist *over a reasonably long period of time,* but they are *not* a manifestation of allergy. Treat them simply, with aspirin, ice or cool cloths, and an antihistamine if the itching is severe. They will get better.

HOME TREATMENT AND THE LAST RESORT:
THE ALLERGIST

In this chapter, I have tried to give you a basic understanding of allergy as it affects children and differs in adults, and to talk about the fallacies that have grown up around it. Once a diagnosis of allergy is either made or seriously suspected, it's up to your physician to provide an ongoing program for the child.

There are, of course, measures you can take yourself. Dry skin may be a forerunner of skin allergy. It is worse in the wintertime and may require lubrication from time to time. Although fancy bath oils work, they are expensive and smelly. Try rubbing the child with mineral oil or petroleum jelly from top to bottom once or twice a week just before he goes to bed. (Do it the night before you change the sheets.) Mineral oil and petroleum jelly, at least, are odorless and inexpensive.

Other manifestations of skin allergy (varying degrees of eczema) may require no treatment if they are mild, simple lubrication if they cause mild discomfort, or specific medication (ointment) if they are troublesome. Consult your physician. But don't forget: If the offending agent is known, avoid it.

Little more need be said about food allergies as they apply to either infants or older children. The avoidance of milk, wheat, and eggs has already been mentioned. In older children, it may be possible for you to isolate specific offending foods and drugs. Obviously, they should be avoided. In these older children, the ingestion of allergic foods (commonly shellfish, citrus fruits and juices, chocolate, and nuts) will frequently cause swelling and hives. Try ice applied to the swollen areas; cornstarch or baking-soda baths to relieve itching. Your doctor can prescribe antihistamine preparations, if these are indicated, and will probably recommend that you keep a supply on hand. But remember —prevention is easier than treatment.

Inhalant allergies are more difficult to treat. It may seem impractical to try to control a child's environment, but in many situations the attempt can be made successfully. For example, if a child's symptoms are worse at night, the environment of his room can be altered by eliminating unnecessary furnishings and providing adequate humidification and clean air. Again, antihistamine preparations may be helpful and should be dispensed at the discretion of your physician. Bronchial asthma probably represents the most severe manifestation of inhalant allergy. This will always require the attention of your physician and possibly of a specialist in allergic diseases.

By calling allergy specialists "the last resort" in the title of this section, I do not mean to deny their usefulness. I refer many patients to them, and am thankful for their help. But I do think too many children go to allergists and get put through a broad series of investigative procedures —and, frequently, a prolonged series of densensitizing injections—that may not really be necessary. A certain amount of allergy can be tolerated without any treatment at all. Simple dry skin and occasional nasal stuffiness probably do not warrant specific treatment. Other symptoms frequently can be controlled by avoidance and environmental measures.

Finally, if, in the opinion of your physician, the symptoms of allergy are severe enough to require a specialist's diagnosis and treatment, the allergist should be consulted. My own criterian for making such a judgment is simple: If the symptoms, inconvenience, and restriction of the allergic child's activities are worse than the anticipated treatment (allergy testing and a series of desensitizing injections), then it is time to treat.

6

Rashes and the Contagious Diseases of Childhood

This chapter deals with *contemporary* common contagious diseases of childhood that are associated with rashes and for which no vaccines are available. Most of the more familiar communicable childhood diseases such as measles and German measles have succumbed to vaccines and no longer need be discussed. I am assuming that your children will be immunized at appropriate ages (see the immunization schedules in Appendix 1). Most of the viral rashes considered here are newly identified and classified, although they've probably always been with us.

COMMON CONTAGIOUS DISEASES

Chicken pox and scarlet fever are actually the only two common contagious diseases of childhood that are left to talk about. Diphtheria, whooping cough, tetanus, and polio are statistical rarities thanks to immunization. And they don't produce rashes. Nor does mumps, although the patient's face swells. And mumps, too, should become rare with the advent of vaccine. Smallpox, of course, has not been seen in the United States since 1949. And both types of measles —the ten-day, or regular, variety (rubeola) and the three-day, or German, measles (rubella)—are fast disappearing now that vaccine is available.

Except for polio, virus vaccines are not given until one year of age. This is because immunity derived from the mother may still be present in the child's bloodstream and prevent the "take" of the vaccine. (See immunization schedule in Appendix 1.) Fortunately this very residual immunity also serves to lessen the severity of the disease if an infant is exposed prior to immunization.

Chicken Pox (Varicella)

The best clue to the diagnosis of chicken pox is exposure, since this is one of the most contagious diseases a child can get. Heed the warning about a case in the classroom, note the date on which the exposure took place, and look for pox in your own child about two weeks later. Although the incubation period can be as short as ten days or as long as twenty days, two weeks is usual.

When one of your children comes down with chicken pox, keep his brothers and sisters (even the infant over three months of age) as far away from him as possible. They will all get chicken pox if they haven't had it before, but the farther away you keep them, the lighter the cases will be.

The rash appears as individual red, pimplelike spots about an eighth of an inch across that quickly turn into tiny, clear blisters. You may have to look carefully for these blisters; they can be quite small, they itch intensely, and may be quickly scratched off. They will then form scabs, which appear a day or two after the blisters. Successive crops of pox appear over the first four or five days of the illness. These are located mostly on the body but also in the scalp and on the face and genitals. In infants and small children, the rash may be particularly profuse in the diaper area. It is sparse on the arms and legs and rare on the palms and soles, but may occur in the mouth, throat, and ears.

Chicken pox is contagious from one day *before* the onset of the rash until all the pox have scabbed and are dry —usually five to seven days after the appearance of the first pox. In the first twenty-four hours it spreads through classrooms of kids, no matter how conscientious the parents. Fortunately, children are not usually very sick with chicken pox. Fever is low-grade (100° to 102° F.) and may be treated with light clothing, aspirin if necessary, and increased liquids. The itching that always goes with the rash will be helped by calamine preparations applied frequently, cornstarch or baking-soda paste or baths, aspirin (yes, aspirin helps itching), or, if necessary, a fancier anti-itch medication that your physician may prescribe. Itching should be treated *through* the scab stage, because scabs that have been scratched off too early are more likely to scar.

Complications can occur in chicken pox. Fever over 103° to 104° F. that lasts more than a few hours, persistent racking cough, unusual sleepiness, severe headache, persistent vomiting, or the appearance of bleeding into the skin (bruising without injury) are all symptoms that should alert you to call your physician.

Shingles, or herpes zoster infection, is a different disease caused by the same virus that causes chicken pox. It rarely occurs in children. Probably as a result of incomplete immunity from a childhood case of chicken pox, the susceptible adult, when reexposed to chicken pox (or another case of shingles in an adult), develops pain in a specific segment on one side of his body or the other (never both). This progresses to a rash, resembling chicken pox, that hurts rather than itches. Shingles does not get complicated and requires only the relief of pain. But you should know that susceptible children can acquire chicken pox from adults with shingles, and vice versa.

Scarlet Fever (Scarlatina)

Scarlet fever is a streptococcal sore throat with a rash. That's all it is. Erythrogenic toxin (red-producing poison) is released, forming a rash of pinhead-sized red dots too numerous to count. These dots give the skin the appearance of a scarlet flush, prominent over the cheeks, chest, abdomen, and, especially, the groin. The dots coalesce (come together) in skin folds, so that normal skin creases look like red lines. The little bumps of the tongue get bigger and redder, producing the appearance of a strawberry or raspberry texture, depending on how much white coating is present between the bumps.

Scarlet fever is important, *not* because of the bad prognosis of prepenicillin days, but because of the necessity for diagnosis and adequate treatment with appropriate antibiotics, preferably penicillin. As a matter of fact, older doctors say that the disease has become much milder in the last half century.

Following the acute illness by ten days to three weeks, there is frequently a peeling of the palms and soles (or even other areas of the skin) that is neither severe nor of clinical consequence. Its only significance is in making a retrospective diagnosis of scarlet fever in a child with a previous history of sore throat and rash who was not treated by a physician. Should this peeling occur, it is probably worth a throat culture, even in an otherwise well child; if the streptococcus is still present, it should be treated. (See Streptococcal Sore Throat in Chapter 2.)

Other Viral Rashes

At least five hundred different viruses have now been isolated that are theoretically capable of producing illness in humans; well over one hundred of them have been known to do so.

Many of the less well known viruses produce fever and sore throat as predominant symptoms. In these cases, streptococcal sore throat must be considered a possibility. I am not convinced, however, that these children need be seen by a doctor. If the child is not very ill, and symptoms can be managed with simple remedies (aspirin, fluids, gargles, and rest), a throat culture can be made by the physician's nurse or office assistant. If the streptococcus is found, the physician can then prescribe an antibiotic. Delaying specific treatment of streptococcal infection for a day or two does not significantly increase the risk of streptococcal complications (i.e., rheumatic fever or nephritis), and the needless use of antibiotics can be avoided.

ECHO [1] and Coxsackie [2] Viruses

If fever and sore throat are accompanied by a rash, the child should be seen by the physician to make or rule out the diagnosis of scarlet fever. The rashes of ECHO and Coxsackie viruses are usually different from that of scarlet fever, but sometimes they are similar and may be confusing. ECHO or Coxsackie viruses are usually the culprits if the streptococcus is not found. Simple home remedies are as effective here as antibiotics, which means the latter need not be used.

Here are some other viral syndromes you may recognize. In a sense, they have replaced the usual common contagious diseases of childhood. Unless otherwise indicated, home remedies are all that is required.

Roseola (Infantum)

This disease is most commonly seen in babies a year old or so, but it may occur any time between six months and two years. The onset of roseola is characterized by sudden appearance of high fever (103° to 105° F.) without any other symptoms. This is apt to persist for two to three days. If the doctor examines the child, he will not find any obvious cause for the fever. At the end of the two- to three-

1. "ECHO" does not mean that the illness is recurrent—it's an acronym. The virus, grown in human tissue culture before it was associated with any specific disease, was therefore assigned the four initials: E for enteric (found in the intestine); C for cytopathogenic (capable of invading cells); H for human (grown in human tissue culture); O for orphan (the researchers didn't know the disease the virus caused).

2. Named after the town in New York where the virus was first identified. At that time, a rare strain was causing temporary paralysis, and Coxsackie was therefore confused with polio—until the patients all recovered.

day period the infant's temperature returns to normal or even goes below normal (97° to 98° F.), and he will become very grouchy and irritable. Finally, a red "measley" rash appears over the face and trunk. The disposition of the child (and his parents) returns to normal; the rash fades in twenty-four hours; and everyone is relieved.

However, there is a possibility of convulsions with this high fever. Fortunately these are usually brief, do not recur, and have no aftereffects. (See Chapter 1 for a discussion of febrile convulsions.)

When the child's fever is at its height, the anxiety of the parents and the desire of the physician to "do something" frequently provoke a decision to treat with antibiotics. The judgment is a difficult one. But then, when the rash finally occurs, the possibility of antibiotic allergy has to be raised. As a result, many children live out their lives with a presumed diagnosis of penicillin allergy. Perhaps some of the newer, safer, and more reliable skin tests for penicillin allergy that are currently being introduced will eliminate this complication.

Boston Exanthem (Fifth Disease)

This virus infection is so named because the first epidemic of it was described in Boston and because it was the fifth of the red-rash contagious diseases to be identified (the first four being regular measles, German measles, scarlet fever, and roseola).

The illness is very mild; frequently, no fever or debilitation occurs at all. The rash, however, is characteristic. On the first day, the cheeks have a bright scarlet flush. On the second day, the flush of the cheeks is replaced by a delicate, lacelike red rash *under* the skin of the *outer sides* of the arms and legs. On the third day this progresses to the trunk and the inner sides of the extremities and then disappears. There is no itching, no treatment, no complication —no worry.

Adeno-Pharyngeal-Conjunctival Fever

This is another sore-throat disease, but the tipoff is the simultaneous appearance of conjunctivitis (inflammation of the eyes with pus). The conjunctivitis may precede the sore throat. Rash has not been associated with this disease, although I suppose conjunctivitis could be considered a rash of the mucous membrane of the eye. (That would at least justify its inclusion in this chapter.) Again, a throat culture may be made to rule out streptococcal infection, but this is not usually necessary when the conjunctivitis occurs.

The important consideration in this disease is the adenoidal swelling. (See Chapter 2 for the relationship between adenoidal swelling and middle-ear infection.) It is helpful to begin a nasal decongestant (nose drops or syrup) when the diagnosis of adeno-pharyngeal-conjunctival fever is made. It may help to prevent a middle-ear infection, especially if the patient has a previous history of ear problems. Many good decongestants are available over the counter. (See Appendix 2.) The eyes need only an occasional wipe with a cotton ball dipped in lukewarm water. The pus will disappear in a few days.

Cold Sores (Fever Blisters)

Call them what you will, these are symptoms of a herpes virus infection and they are extremely common. Mentioned here because of their tendency to recur, they are frequently confused with impetigo.

The primary infection usually occurs in infants and small toddlers and is accompanied by a fever. The mouth becomes full of canker sores—whitish ulcers of various sizes, surrounded by reddened areas all over the mucous membrane of the mouth. Quite painful. They usually heal without benefit of specific treatment, although the encouragement of fluids is important. The child usually doesn't want to eat or drink because his mouth hurts when he does. And he won't thank you for anything spicy, salty, citrusy, or carbonated.

Thereafter, some children will get more than their share of *recurrent* cold sores, clusters of little blisters that appear somewhere between the lower lip and chin. (Impetigo's usual site is on the upper lip, closer to the nostril.) They appear after colds or other illnesses with fever, but sometimes they appear for no good reason at all.

Although cold sores can become secondarily infected, they usually do not. They blister, weep, and scab, then finally dry up and disappear. This takes seven to ten days.

The treatment is symptomatic and conservative. Your pharmacist will have a number of patent medicines that may help. Old-fashioned camphor ice or lip balm is as good as any. Be encouraged by the fact that febrile illnesses and colds diminish in frequency and intensity as your child grows older. Cold sores or fever blisters usually follow the same pattern.

7

Problems of the Newborn, Real and Imaginary

Most life-threatening congenital abnormalities show up in the first few days of life. That is why pediatricians like to keep newborns in the hospital for three or four days. It is true that with the high cost of hospitalization there is a tendency for women to go home very quickly. But the newborn does need some observation, and if he is allowed to remain in the hospital for a few days, his parents will have greater assurance (statistically, at least) that what they notice at home will probably be normal.

On the other hand, the normal newborn has many physical characteristics that differ from those of older children and adults. Let's try to sort out some of these differences.

JAUNDICE

Jaundice is a yellow pigmentation in the skin that occurs frequently in newborns for a variety of reasons and may or may not be serious. Problems arising from jaundice will be investigated before the newborn leaves the hospital. My intention here is to explain how jaundice works.

Unborn babies live in an atmosphere in which less oxygen is available to them than in the outside world. In order that their tissues receive adequate oxygen, their blood is thickened with millions of extra red blood cells. After birth, when a higher oxygen concentration is available, these extra blood cells will frequently make the newly born infant look lobster-red. But since these "extra" red blood cells are no longer needed, they begin to break down. This process releases hemoglobin, which is rapidly transformed chemically to a substance called bilirubin. Bilirubin is yellow. Normally, the liver further processes bilirubin so that it can be excreted from the body via the kidneys and the gastrointestinal tract. But if the liver is slightly immature, and if the amount of bilirubin that needs to be processed is large, then bilirubin may accumulate in the blood and diffuse into tissues and skin, where it is observed as jaundice.

When this happens, the jaundice is usually not severe and causes no harm. Your physician will be on the lookout for jaundice, and if it occurs, he will try to ascertain its cause, measure its intensity (through laboratory tests), watch for possible conditions (liver problems, blood-type incompatibilities, etc.) that could increase the jaundice to toxic levels, and decide what treatment (if any) is appropriate.

Sometimes jaundice does not reach its highest level in the newborn for the better part of a week. Let this, then, help to underline the importance of the newborn infant's initial stay in the hospital for a period of observation. It should not be cut short for financial or emotional reasons.

ANATOMY PECULIAR TO THE NEWBORN

The Head

In order to make it through the birth canal, the head of a newborn has to be malleable. The skull, therefore, is not solid like an eggshell, but rather more like the covering of an armadillo, with movable plates of bone (sheathed in a casing of skin and membrane) that are capable of being molded by external forces. Sometimes head molding is all too obvious for a few days or even weeks, but it eventually smooths out.

One rather large lump or "goose egg" may persist, usually on one side (rarely on both) and toward the back of the head. This is probably a *cephalhematoma,* a collection of blood and fluid under the scalp that is formed at the time of delivery. Although it sometimes lasts for weeks or even months, it never causes problems, and it subsides spontaneously. Other by-products of delivery are bruises or forceps marks on the face, or large red spots in the white of the eyes. These, too, will resolve with time.

When you bring your baby home, his eyes may still be swollen and may fill with yellow mucus from time to time. This is a chemical conjunctivitis caused by the silver nitrate that was instilled in his eyes immediately after birth to prevent infection. The outpouring of white blood cells kills any bacteria that may be present. This, too, usually clears within a few days, and all you need to do is keep the eyes clean. A cotton ball dipped in lukewarm water (neither has to be sterile) will do the job.

Occasionally, after the conjunctivitis clears, one eye or the other will tear from time to time. The tears usually will be clear, although now and then they may contain mucus for a few days. This is almost certainly due to an *obstructed tear duct* resulting from the chemical conjunctivitis. The condition usually clears spontaneously some time during the first year. It should be brought to the attention of your physician when you see him for a routine checkup, but it does not require a special visit. Even when mucus is noted, no special medication (other than the cotton-ball technique just described) is necessary.

If the tearing does not stop spontaneously by the end of the first year, the duct may have to be probed. Your physician will make the decision at the appropriate time. Don't be surprised if he tells you that the procedure will require a brief hospital admission for general anesthesia. This is delicate work, and a one-year-old just won't stay still for it. Be assured that the procedure is not complicated.

You may notice white patches of material that remain long after a milk feed on your baby's tongue and inside the cheeks and lips. If you try to remove them and find that they won't scrape off, he almost certainly has *thrush,* an infection caused by a yeastlike organism called monilia or candida. The odds are that this condition was acquired from his mother's vagina during delivery and lay dormant for a few weeks before appearing in the baby's mouth. (Monilia is a common vaginal inhabitant, especially during pregnancy.) A call to your physician will provide medication that will clear up the infection readily. And the mother should consult her obstetrician, too, to be sure that *her* infection is cleared up.

Cradle cap can be thought of as severe dandruff. It is caused by insufficient stimulation of the scalp. Most infants' heads are overprotected to such a degree (the soft spot, a place in the front of the top of the head where four plates of bone will eventually fuse, is sacrosanct) that they are inadequately cleansed and stimulated. Their hairbrushes have the impact of a feather duster. If you want to prevent cradle cap, give the baby's scalp a good scrub with a washcloth and soap a couple of times a week. And if you see evidence of crusting and discoloration of the scalp, you're not scrubbing vigorously enough. Use your fingernails, a bristle brush, or a fine comb, and get in there and scrape! He may not like it, but it only takes a few minutes and he'll be a lot better off for it. And don't be afraid of the soft spot. You can't hurt him.

The Chest

A newborn's nipples will sometimes excrete a few drops of white liquid during the first week or so. This can occur in both girls and boys. It is caused by the withdrawal of high levels of female hormones from the baby's bloodstream immediately following birth, and it will stop within a few days. The nipples should be left alone. Don't squeeze them to see if there's any fluid left. Even if the breasts themselves seem slightly enlarged or swollen, they will recede if they are left alone. On the other hand, single-breast swelling—especially if accompanied by redness, streaking, tenderness, irritability, or fever—should be brought to your physician's attention. It means the same thing in the baby that it means in the mother, a breast abscess.

One thing more about the chest. At the bottom of the breastbone (sternum), there is a small triangular bone called the *xiphoid*. If an infant is thin, this bone sometimes sticks up and out. Because of its proximity to the abdomen, and because to some, "anything sticking out of the abdomen is a hernia," people worry. Don't. It will straighten out.

The Abdomen

Most infants come home from the hospital with a remnant of the umbilical cord still attached to the belly button (umbilicus). This will fall off in a week or two. Keep it clean, and follow your physician's instructions for routine care. A drop or two of blood on the diaper or shirt is perfectly normal. No bandage, binding, or tape is required.

After the cord comes off, the umbilicus should dry up within a few days. If it doesn't, an *umbilical granuloma* may be present. This is a little nubbin of tissue *in* the umbilicus at the junction of old cord and new skin. It's almost as if the tissue can't make up its mind whether to live or die, and so it weeps. This can be easily remedied when you visit the doctor for the baby's first checkup. A special visit is not necessary.

Umbilical hernias (the belly button protrudes) do occur from time to time but are no cause for alarm. The overwhelming majority will reduce themselves and close up spontaneously by the second or third year. They do not need the help of belly bands, band-aids, adhesive, coins strapped to the abdomen, or any other device. They almost never cause trouble in childhood. The only problems are a cosmetic one for the infant and anxiety for the parents, neither of which is a good reason for surgery. If your baby has an umbilical hernia, leave it alone. It will take care of itself.

During infancy hernias may also occur in the groin, on one or both sides. Both boys and girls get them. They are called *inguinal hernias* and appear as lumps, olive- to plum-sized, usually when the infant is crying. They can be pushed back easily when the infant stops crying, and they often reduce themselves spontaneously—although usually they will reappear from time to time. Under normal circumstances they cause no discomfort and can be brought to the attention of your physician at the infant's next regularly scheduled visit. However, if the lump cannot be pushed back or does not reduce itself, if it gets tender or swollen, if the child becomes quite irritable, and especially if he starts to vomit, you should call your physician without delay. Strangulation of the hernia is a possibility.

Many physicians recommend surgery when such a hernia is discovered. This is not an emergency procedure unless the possibility of strangulation of the hernia is imminent, but the odds are that surgery will be required sooner or later. "Sooner" will mean greater peace of mind for the parents and the physician and will prevent the possibility of inadvertent strangulation at some future date. Considering that it is the bowel that usually is being herniated in boys and the ovary in girls, most physicians do not want to risk putting off surgery.

Many surgeons prefer to operate on both sides, even though only one is herniated. They cite a large incidence of recurrence of the hernia on the opposite side at a later date and feel that if both sides are operated on at one time, additional hospitalization may be prevented. This is especially true for boys. Another school of thought has it that surgery allows the possibility (although remote) of injury to the genital support structures that pass through the groin. On this basis, surgery can be justified only on the obviously affected side. I urge you to accept the advice of your physician and surgeon when you make your decision. Be reassured, however, that either procedure is usually simple, safe, and satisfactory in outcome.

The Genitals

Girl babies frequently have a vaginal discharge when they get home from the hospital. It may be thick and whitish, and it may even be a little bloody. This is a hormone-withdrawal phenomenon, similar to the one in which fluid is excreted from an infant's nipples. It will clear up shortly.

Sometime, later in the first year, the baby girl's vaginal lips may fuse in varying degrees; this is called labial fusion. It may appear to be so complete that you wonder if there is enough of an opening to allow urination. There is. Again, there are schools of thought that say "treat it" and others that say "leave it alone." My feeling is that so long as the baby is able to urinate comfortably, the situation is best left alone. Later in childhood, the fusion will open up by itself under normal hormonal influence. You may feel better if your physician separates the labia, but you will probably have to apply a hormone cream to them intermittently to keep them open. I think it's more trouble than it's worth.

Boys will frequently get a small irritation or ulceration on the very tip of the penis. (This is really a form of diaper rash, but since it may occur as an isolated spot, without any other sign of rash, it is discussed here separately.) It occurs more often in circumcized boys. All you need to do is keep the area meticulously clean and apply some bland and soothing ointment frequently. Soft paper diaper liners will also help and should be tried in difficult cases.

Now that so many people are opposed to surgical procedures that neither cure a disease nor correct a defect, I suppose we should take another look at the pros and cons of *circumcision*. The proponents will tell you it is an innocuous procedure that the infant hardly feels. (The complication rate from the procedure itself is minuscule.) They say that circumcision cures phimosis (inability of the foreskin to be retracted) in the newborn and prevents it in adults. And, finally, they claim that it lowers the rate of cancer of the cervix in women—smegma (secretions that collect under the foreskin) may be cancer-producing.

Opponents of circumcision will argue that even the minuscule risk of complications is not justified. They say that most newborns have phimosis (this is true) and that there is no need for the foreskin to be retractable until much later in life. Infection is hardly ever seen in children, and phimosis of the newborn cures itself with the coming of the erection phenomenon. (This occurs in the first few years of life.) They say that few adults ever require circumcision and that even fewer of them would if they were taught proper hygiene. And they feel that better hygienic measures (rather than circumcision) could help to reduce the incidence of cervical cancer.

These are most of the medical arguments. I won't go into the emotional ones. When asked, I recommend circumcision, mostly to avoid future problems or future *concern* over problems.

The testicles usually present no problem. Sometimes one or both of them seem quite large, and, at a routine visit, your physician may make the diagnosis of *hydrocoele* (water sac) around the testis. Most hydrocoeles disappear after a few months and are no cause for concern. But babies with hydrocoeles have a greater incidence of inguinal hernia, so you will want to be alert to any problems in the groin area. Notwithstanding the previous discussion of hernias, the presence of hydrocoeles is *not,* by itself, a reason for surgery during the newborn period or for some time thereafter.

Similarly, *undescended testicles* may require surgery later in childhood but should not concern you in the newborn. Much depends on whether one or both testes are undescended, whether they can be located, what they feel like, and the child's age. There are too many variables involved for me to attempt to make a definitive statement here. Your physician is the person best qualified to make the decision concerning surgery.

The Skin

Most newborn infants are dressed too warmly. Their skin responds with *miliaria* (obstructed sweat glands), white dots over the face in the areas usually associated with perspiration, and with *prickly heat* (red dots, single and multiple, and more widespread, appearing on the head, neck, and shoulders). Although a few infants have problems with temperature regulation in the first few days of life, most do not. They want to be as warm or as cool as you do. And remember, when they're crying, they expend as much energy as you might running around the block wearing an undershirt, diaper, plastic pants, shirt, nightshirt, flannel receiving blanket, and a woolen cover. Imagine!

Birthmarks come in all sizes, shapes, and colors. Only a few (and rare ones at that) concern us. The flat, pink ones on the upper eyelids, lower forehead, and back of the head and neck will go away. The large, flat, bluish ones of varying shapes on the lower back will disappear, too. Brown moles and tan, flat, oval, well-marked areas (café-au-lait spots) are probably there to stay and will cause no harm. The doctor will keep track of them during routine examinations.

Hemangiomas appear anywhere on the body and are

lumps that look like small strawberries. They usually appear *after* birth and enlarge to various sizes during the first few months of life. They become raised, red, and soft, and can cause quite a bit of concern in the uninformed. Most of them will disappear totally *if* they are left alone. It is a shame to risk scarring a child by surgery, dry ice, acid, or injection when the treatment is unnecessary. And if you are concerned that your child's hemangioma may be one that won't disappear, remember that the odds are twenty to one that it will. They usually don't get injured or bleed, and if surgery is necessary, it will probably be easier to handle when the child is older and more cooperative. The procedure is also less extensive if performed later on.

DIAPER RASH

There are essentially three causes of diaper rash, and most cases result from any one of a combination of these.

Inadequate Cleansing

Before you get angry with me, read on. I am not suggesting that you are a negligent parent, only that your baby may have more delicate skin than most. His skin just can't tolerate constant wetness and fecal soiling. Once a rash appears, you should do everything you can to minimize the insult to the skin of his diaper area:

1.   Eliminate rubber and plastic pants. You want to let the moisture out, not keep it in. If you use disposable diapers, take the plastic off.

2.   Put double diapers on him during the day and triple

diapers at night. The more moisture the diaper absorbs, the less there will be next to the skin.

3. Wash the diaper area with soap and water at every diaper change (even if he's only wet). Rinse well.

4. Use baby powder and a bland, soothing ointment alternately at each diaper change (see Appendix 2). Adjust this schedule so that the ointment is used prenap and pre-sleep. But don't use it all the time. It takes too much scrubbing to get off, which may injure the baby's skin.

5. Give the baby extra fluids so that the urine will be less concentrated, and slow down on fruits if he's having too many stools.

These measures will cure most diaper rash. The intensity of the treatment may then be varied depending on what the healed skin can tolerate.

Ammoniacal Dermatitis

Some infants are great ammonia producers. Actually, it's urea, a precursor of ammonia that breaks down to ammonia later. The most obvious symptom of this condition is the intense smell of ammonia present when the infant has his first diaper change in the morning. At that time, the skin is apt to be fiery red and tender, just as if it had been scalded with hot water. Follow the treatment outlined in the above checklist, with an emphasis on increasing liquid intake in order to reduce the concentration of the urine. In addition, if you wash your own diapers, add a half cup of white vinegar to the last rinse. (Vinegar is a mild solution of acetic acid that retards the conversion of urea to free ammonia.) Finally, if these measures don't suffice, ask your physician to prescribe a medication that will alter the chemistry of the urine so that less ammonia is produced.

Thrush of the Skin

Earlier I talked about thrush in an infant's mouth. Actually the infection can go all the way through the gastrointestinal tract, come out the anus, and infect the skin of the diaper area. Spreading out from the anus, a mass of violaceous red pimples may coalesce into a fiery red rash that has sharply demarcated borders. This can cover part or all of the skin in the diaper area. If you have done all the things listed above to eliminate simple and ammoniacal dermatitis without success, and if the rash fits this description, there is a very good chance that thrush is the problem. This diagnosis is almost certain if mother has a troublesome vaginal discharge or if the baby has thrush in his mouth. Your physician ought to see this rash so that he can diagnose it properly and treat it as he thinks necessary. And the baby's mother should see her obstetrician.

BEHAVIOR PECULIAR TO THE NEWBORN

Newborn infants sleep a lot, sometimes as much as twenty hours a day when they first come home. As the months go by, they want to spend more time awake, want to be played with, and want to enjoy the new world around them. But an infant that stays sleepy month after month may have a problem.

Newborns startle, shudder, twitch, and shake. This probably represents an untrained and spontaneously reactive central nervous system. The behavior is normal and soon changes. On the other hand, uncontrolled, generalized spasms of the entire body, especially if accompanied by high fever, breath-holding, or turning blue, may mean the baby is having a convulsion (see discussion of febrile convulsions in Chapter 1). Call your doctor immediately!

Newborn infants spit up and vomit from time to time. (I consider spitting up the same as "a little vomiting.") They do this because they are overfed, underburped, positioned poorly, or fed too fast—to give a few reasons. This is normal. If an infant vomits consistently, meal after meal, he may have a problem. Call your physician.

Newborns like to suck. It is their most satisfactory form of gratification. Their need to suck frequently goes beyond their need to eat. Often they will awaken an hour after a feed and seem hungry (putting their hands in their mouths, and so forth). If you offer a second feed, they may take half an ounce or so and then go back to sleep. They weren't really hungry for that half an ounce, they just wanted to suck. This is where the pacifier comes in.

If you don't believe in using a pacifier, stop and think a minute. What you probably disapprove of is the sight of a toddler walking around with a pacifier stuck in his mouth like a plug. I agree with you. But sometime during the second half of the baby's first year, you will note that the pacifier no longer pacifies him. *That's* the time to take it away.

Let me give you one example of the improper use of a pacifier. The doctor gives the baby a shot, he starts to cry, and mother shoves the pacifier in his mouth. *Wrong!* He has been hurt, and he's entitled to cry. Pick him up and love him a little, but don't shove the plug in.

Note that most pacifiers have a nipple, a shield, and a ring. Take the ring off. He may catch a finger in the ring, inadvertently pull the pacifier out of his mouth, and howl!

Breast-fed newborns have peculiar *bowel movements,* by any adult standard. When they first come home from the hospital, they usually have a bowel movement every time they feed. This is apt to be watery, seedy, and golden yellow in color. It's a mess, but it's normal. Somewhere between the third and sixth week, however, the movements slow up and firm up. A new pattern emerges that looks like constipation but isn't. They are apt to have one bowel movement every three to seven days. The stool is large, yellow, and pasty, not hard. And it may take all day to pass. They don't really have any trouble moving it, although they may grunt and groan for hours. It may take the form of three or four partial movements over the course of a day, but it is really one big evacuation. Then they are finished for a few days. The only way that I can explain this phenomenon is to postulate that breast milk is so well utilized that there is precious little waste.

In summary, then, the newborn is a different being from the adult. Much of what he is and does is abnormal for adults but normal for him. And short of throwing him around too much, you can't hurt him. As a matter of fact, I believe that more harm comes to him from too much care and concern than from too little. Common sense should get you through most of the problem situations that arise.

8

Other Common Skin Problems

Other rashes bring children into doctors' offices in tremendous numbers—possibly because they are so obvious, but probably because children get so many of them. Although there are rare and mysterious rashes, a few common skin conditions account for the majority of these office visits.

Let's leave what is esoteric for the dermatologists and consider *pediatric* dermatology. These are rashes that you can diagnose and treat (at least the second time around). They tend to be either chronic or recurrent, so you will probably get more than one crack at them. And you should try. The odds are that you'll be successful; even if you're not, little harm will be done. They frequently get better by themselves, given a little time; and you can always see the doctor later without your child having suffered.

One cardinal principle should be followed in managing all skin conditions: cleanliness is essential. Infection is an ever-present hazard in any area where a child has broken skin. Warm water, soap, and a washcloth will do much to prevent infection, remove scabs and old skin, bring the body's own healing agents to the area (by means of the stimulation and warmth of the wash), and provide a receptive surface on which to apply whatever local healing medication may be indicated.

POISON IVY, OAK, AND SUMAC

Certainly the most common rash in my area (Connecticut) is poison ivy/oak/sumac. But it is indigenous to most of the country, and is truly a rash for all seasons. The plants stay alive all year long (although they are more abundant in the summer and fall), so that children can contact them in any season.

The rash, which itches intensely, appears hours to days after contact. It looks like little pimples and blisters distributed across the skin in an erratic fashion that coincides with the way the contact was made. Thus, if a leaf brushed across the forearm or leg, there will be a streak of pimples or blisters following the path of the leaf. If a child was walking through a patch of poison ivy or rummaging through it with his hands looking for something, it will be *all over* the hands or feet. Here, so much of the skin will be affected that the little blisters will come together to form large ones that are incapacitating and quite painful. Boys frequently get a small patch of the rash near or on their genitals. (They find it convenient to relieve themselves behind a tree or bush when they have the plant oil on their fingers; it transfers readily.)

In the fall months, children will occasionally get a fine flush of poison ivy uniformly distributed over the face. This may be related to the burning of leaves that have poison ivy in them. Apparently the smoke contains fine particulate matter to which the plant oil still adheres, and this is deposited on the face.

Contaminated clothing—especially sneakers, caps, and other gear not frequently washed—is another source of contact. Keep this in mind in recurrent cases. Finally, if a child gets poison ivy when he hasn't been out in the woods for weeks, cast a suspicious look at the family dog or cat. An animal will frequently walk through the foliage and get the oil on its hair. If a child fondles the animal shortly thereafter, he can get a good case. This source is particularly likely when the rash appears in large patches on the face and neck.

How is poison ivy spread? Let's clear up a misconception right now. *Only* the oil of the plant is contagious. The fluid contained within poison ivy blisters is not contagious and therefore does not spread the pimples or blisters. Once your child has had a good wash and all the oil is removed, the rash cannot spread. Sometimes it seems to spread, but this is because it comes out slowly, in successive crops, or because there is continual reexposure to the plant oil. The *only* way the child can spread the disease is by spreading the plant oil. Therefore, once you know that a child has just come into contact with poison ivy, the faster you wash him thoroughly, the less plant oil will penetrate the skin and the less poison ivy will develop. Scrub first.

Prevention, of course, is preferable to treatment. This can be accomplished by keeping children out of the poison ivy or by getting rid of it when it appears on limited tracts of land. This approach works with younger children, who are more readily controlled and don't wander too far.

In the case of older children, who can't or won't keep

away from the stuff, desensitization may be considered. There are oral preparations of highly diluted solutions of poison ivy extract that are given in increasing doses in an attempt to desensitize the child and build up a tolerance to the plant oil. Many physicians think that the oral preparations don't work very well and that a series of shots does a better job. There is little evidence to favor or disprove either approach. My feeling on all desensitization treatments in children is that the intensity of the treatment must be justified by the severity of the disease.

Simple measures in the treatment of poison ivy include keeping the area clean and soothing the itch with calamine lotion preparations. The large blisters that often develop between the fingers and toes may be quite uncomfortable. They can be cleaned thoroughly, and "popped" with a sterilized needle or scissors point. An antibiotic ointment should then be applied (available over the counter) to retard infection and prevent the bandage (a wrapping of sterile gauze) from sticking. Aspirin will help the itching.

If a child is quite uncomfortable despite these simple measures, call your doctor. He can order more specific medicines, sometimes without seeing the child, to ease the discomfort. In severe cases, he can administer stronger drugs that will clear the condition more rapidly and provide significant comfort in the process.

ECZEMA

The skin's most common manifestation of allergy is eczema. It comes in a variety of sizes and shapes depending on the place on the skin at which it erupts, the age group, and the time of year. Experience has shown that your child's eczema will probably require the attention of your doctor sooner or later; sooner is preferable. There are many factors that will have to be considered, medications that will have to be tried, and dietary changes that may be necessary. It is my purpose here to alert you to some of the symptoms and the appearance of eczema and to answer some of the questions you may have about the disease.

In infants, eczema is most apt to occur on the cheeks as a shiny, red, flat, rather patchy rash that itches. It varies in size and shape, appears on one cheek or both, and changes color, shape, and size from day to day. If scratched continuously, it weeps; and when the wetness dries, it scabs. Other common locations for the same type of rash are behind the ears, around the navel, and under the diaper. It frequently appears in elongated stretches under the edge of the diaper, across the abdomen, in the groin, and around the backs of the legs. Sometimes it is the result of a chronic irritation where plastic or rubber pants touch the skin. The rash under the diaper is usually dry and thickened rather than moist and scabbed. Perhaps that is because it is less accessible and is not scratched as much as exposed areas. Nevertheless, the infant may dig at these spots during diaper changes, and long scratch marks frequently result.

Mild eczema that doesn't weep and doesn't seem to bother the child can be treated simply by keeping it clean and applying a bland ointment. It will come and go and probably require no further treatment. If it is bothersome to the baby, call your doctor.

More severe eczema, the chronic variety, is usually found in older children inside the bend of the arm and behind the knee. It will certainly require your physician's help.

Again, here are some general points worth remembering:

1. Since these areas are continually being scratched, they must be kept clean. It's a good idea, too, to keep the fingernails short, smooth, and well scrubbed.

2. In the course of any one day, the constant admonitions to "stop scratching" fall on deaf ears—especially after you've repeated it twenty or thirty times. Don't nag—you'll both be better off for it.

3. A favorite saying of some dermatologists is that eczema is made worse by winter, wool, and worry. Eliminate the wool, and manage the winter and worry as best you can. The contributing factors in winter are overdressing and lack of humidity. These, at least, you can do something about.

4. Ointments and salves are commonly used in the treatment of eczema. Follow your doctor's instructions exactly. Cortisone-containing preparations should be used *only* as prescribed. Even more important, they should never be used for other, undiagnosed rashes. They work well when used as prescribed, but they *can do harm* when used on rashes that are infected.

Coal-tar preparations have been used successfully to treat eczema for many years. They still have a place in treatment, especially in the most chronic cases, and are much less expensive than cortisone. They generally work well when used in a thin layer, applied frequently (up to six times per day), for as many days as it takes to clear up the eczema. The ointment should then be stopped completely and saved for another concentrated series of applications. But don't fiddle with it (don't apply a little now and then; it loses its effectiveness).

Less Common Forms of Eczema

Many children and adults have unusually *dry skin*. Their skin is so dry, in fact, that it may scale in the winter or have many little bumps or pimples that itch along the outer surface of the arms and legs. It is generally believed that this is a manifestation of eczema or an eczemoid rash, although allergy does not seem to play a role. Nothing really seems to cure this condition, although skin lubricants help, especially in cold weather. Dermatologists recommend selective bathing during winter, hitting the areas that need it the most and sparing the outer surfaces of the arms and legs as much as possible.

One treatment that works fairly well is to cover the child from head to toe with a thin layer of mineral oil, once or twice a week, at bedtime, and allow it to remain on all night. This form of treatment is least expensive and the least likely to produce reactions to the ingredients (as may happen with fancier lotions), and it seems to work as well as other lubricants.

Toe eczema usually occurs in older children and adults. The significance of this problem is that it is frequently misdiagnosed as athlete's foot. Both conditions involve cracked and peeling areas of the toes, are intensely itchy, and occur most commonly in feet that perspire a great deal. But here the similarity ends. The first clue is found in the season of the year. Athlete's foot is a summer disease; eczema prefers the winter. The diagnosis is made when the eczema does not respond to antifungus athlete's foot preparations. The treatment of toe eczema may require only the elimination of rubber boots and nylon socks (or tights). The severity of the condition seems to be so closely correlated with how much the feet perspire that these measures may be enough. The child should also be encouraged to go barefoot or wear sandals at home and to change to sandals or thin cloth sneakers at school.

Reference has been made to swimmer's ear, an infection of the ear canal that occurs commonly in children whose ears are often wet in summer. When the usual treatment fails, or when the swimmer's ear persists into the fall and winter, wonder about *ear canal eczema*. It's hard to determine whether this is true primary eczema or an allergic reaction to the local medication used to treat the swimmer's ear, but I have seen the condition recur in winter when there was no intervening exposure to swimmer's ear medicine. Especially in an allergic child, wintertime swimmer's ear is eczema until proven otherwise.

This condition will require your physician to make the diagnosis, clean the ear out when necessary, and prescribe the appropriate ear drops. Consult him when your treatment of "swimmer's ear" fails.

IMPETIGO AND SKIN INFECTION

This is another example of a condition that used to strike terror into the hearts of parents in the preantibiotic era, but is now easily managed.

Impetigo is characterized by clusters of pimples or blisters that are infected, usually in or around one or both nostrils and extending down toward the upper lip. The child frequently picks at them and then scratches other areas of his body, planting the infection in the scratch. New infections then crop up in various locations, all resembling the original infection of the face.

Actually, this infection can be treated like other skin infections. The infecting agent is usually the streptococcus (see more below) or the staphylococcus, and both are usually susceptible to treatment with antibiotics administered either locally or by mouth. In the milder cases, local treatment at home is adequate. If that doesn't work, and the spread of infection seems out of control, you'll need your doctor's help.

Even before treatment, here is a word about prevention: Skin infections are most common in the summer months, probably because more of the skin is exposed and the skin surface is broken more frequently (bug bites, bruises and scratches, poison ivy). In addition, the warm weather enhances the ability of the bacteria to stay alive, and children get together at beaches, pools, and playgrounds and spread the infection among themselves. And they don't use much soap during the summertime; they swim instead. Here, then, is a plea for more than an occasional summertime scrub (use a washcloth) and for more shampoos (look for ticks if you live in an appropriate area of the country) and manicures. You'll really cut down on skin infection.

Impetigo becomes scabbed. Because the bacteria live under the scabs, the scabs have to be removed. Frequent warm soaks (twenty minutes of soaking every two hours) followed by gentle soapy scrubs will remove scabs in a day or so. This should be followed by the application of an over-the-counter antibiotic ointment.

Do not use band-aids. Adhesive applied to the skin provides a nice warm shelter in which the bacteria can multiply. And when the adhesive is pulled off, the outer layer of dead skin frequently comes off with it, providing multiple new portals of entry for more bacteria. If you must cover the infection, use gauze wrapped around the extremities (or a large gauze square if it is on the body) so that the adhesive is as far away from the infection as possible.

Sometimes infection is injected under the skin, either by a puncture wound or by a splinter or other foreign body. In this situation, the child will probably get a boil or abscess, rather than impetigo. The infection goes deep, rather than spreading out superficially. The principles of treatment are the same, but the technique varies a little. You have to bring moist heat to the area as often as possible. The moisture keeps the surface soft and free from scabs that might close the entry point of the infection. The heat marshals blood to the general area, which brings with it the cellular elements of the body that fight infection. The battle between the bacteria and the body destroys tissue and produces pus that *must* be allowed to drain. If the portal of entry is still open, the pus will drain spontaneously. If not, the boil or abscess may have to be drained surgically. Surgical drainage is usually indicated when pain stops the child from normal activities, when fever appears, or when no progress has been made in two to three days of good soaking treatment. Often, however, this can be prevented by frequent hot soaks.

You must still pay attention to the surface around the deep infection, especially if pus is continually draining. Keep it meticulously clean, avoid using adhesive, and apply an antibiotic ointment. These measures will all be helpful.

Local infections can and should be handled locally most of the time. But when you can't seem to make any progress in impetigo, when new areas crop up despite your scrubs, when the infection in the nostril persists beyond a few days, when the area around the nostril, face, and/or lip swells and becomes tender, call the doctor. If the infection occurs following recent exposure to someone with a streptococcal sore throat, or if, during the time that you're treating the skin infection, the child or anyone in the house comes down with a sore throat, call the doctor. Impetigo can be caused by the streptococcus, and there are always potential complications with strep. If some red streaking develops, leading away from the area, or if the child develops pain or tenderness in the appropriate lymph glands (in the groin if the infection is on the leg, in the armpit if it is on the arm, under the chin or in front of the ear if it is on the face), call the doctor. And, finally, if the patient develops fever and becomes sick while he has a local skin infection, by all means call the doctor. He can administer appropriate antibiotics and clear the infection readily. And you will not have lost anything.

ACNE

Like the common cold, acne never killed anybody, and so no one worries very much about it—except the kids who have it. Actually, acne is a complex problem, requiring a multidisciplinary approach. Acne is usually most evident in teenagers, but may begin a few years earlier and last many years longer. Heredity, environment, nutrition, hygiene, hormones, fashion—these are all factors that play a role. And there are certainly unanswered questions about acne that make its treatment very difficult.

As is true of so many medical problems, the more mysterious the cause, the greater the variety of medical treatments advocated. Without taking a stand on the merits or inadequacies of more sophisticated methods of treatment, I want to cover some of the basics of good skin care in acne.

The acned face is excessively oily, and the oil plays a role in plugging sweat glands and pores. Dirt, which clings more easily to an oily surface than to a smooth one, provides the "black" for blackheads. Dirt and infection go hand in hand, and many pimples and blemishes become infected. All these factors add up to the importance of keeping the face and other affected areas as clean as possible. In my book, this means hot water, a washcloth and soap, and a five-minute scrub at least three times a day. If the back is involved, and it frequently is, a back brush is essential.

The observation that acne is better in the summer has prompted the use of the sun lamp for year-round treatment. It helps, but must be used with care. The eyes *must* be protected by goggles, and children, even teenagers, should *never* be allowed to use the lamp alone. Too many of them fall asleep and get badly burned. The lamp should be twenty-four inches away from the face. Limit the first exposure to one minute. The exposure time can then be lengthened daily in one-minute increments, depending on how things go. The desired effect is mild redness and subsequent light peeling.

I'm afraid that hair length definitely plays a role in acne. I have never seen acne clear on the back of a girl who wears her hair long and loose. I have never seen acne clear on the forehead of a girl or boy who wears bangs. Unfortunately, in this last case, a vicious cycle is set in motion because the hair is used to hide the pimples. Whether the hair acts as a blanket, a dirt filter, or an oil can, it makes acne worse. Teenagers should be told this, and then given their choice.

There are some recent advances in the treatment of acne that appear to be helpful in specific situations and that should be mentioned here. High doses of vitamin A taken orally have proved useful in some cases. The dose should be prescribed by your physician. A newer preparation, vitamin A acid, shows great promise as a local treatment, but its use is still under investigation. Girls with menstrual irregularities whose doctors put them on hormones have found that their acne has cleared as a result.

Finally, I can't leave the discussion of acne without considering treatment with antibiotics. This is one of my pet peeves, and I hope it will become one of yours.

Many dermatologists advocate the use of antibiotics taken by mouth for acne. Apparently they can produce a dramatic alleviation of infected blemishes. I am sure this is justified in certain cases. But there are children who take antibiotics for months and even years at a time, and I wonder what the protracted use of these drugs does to their internal organs. I have seen at least one critically ill teenager who was suffering from a massive superinfection, the overgrowth of a yeastlike organism that had been allowed to thrive internally because antibiotics had worked to remove normal bacterial growth from his body's environment. I do *not* think that antibiotics should be prescribed for minimal acne or for long periods of time (more than a few weeks); and I do *not* think that children should be allowed to renew their prescriptions at will or to take the medication whenever *they* think they need it.

WARTS

Warts are virus infections and are not dangerous. That much we know about warts, and that's about all we know. Where do they come from? Why do some children get them and others not? Are they contagious? Why do children get them more often than adults? Why do they disappear spontaneously in some children? Why does treatment sometimes work and sometimes have no effect? What's the best treatment?

Huckleberry Finn used the fluid from a hollowed-out tree stump, collected at midnight and mixed with cat's fur and owl feathers. Some of my patients' mothers claim great success with raw hamburger meat applied three times a day. More scientific measures include dermabrasion (a fancy word for using a pumice stone), treatment with acids of varying strengths, surgery, electrical desiccation, X- radiation, ultrasonics, diathermy, vaccination with smallpox vaccine, autosuggestion, and even hypnosis.

All of which suggests that we really don't know what we're doing in treating them. Since the prognosis is so good, you might as well try handling warts yourself. Here are some methods you can follow with a reasonable chance of success.

Of all the possible treatments of warts, autosuggestion is probably the least harmful. Try wishing those warts away. If your child is old enough, give him a rabbit's foot. Send him looking for four-leaf clovers, throw pennies in the well. But do it seriously—that may make the difference.

The second treatment can be combined with the first. Ignore them! They don't exist; you're not worried about them; they really don't bother the patient. Bury your head in the sand; they may go away.

Sometimes warts bleed a little (bleeding can be stopped with pressure, or a styptic pencil). Sometimes they get in the way when the child is writing (especially arithmetic problems and spelling). Here the pumice stone may be helpful, or a mild ointment containing 5 percent salicylic acid. Both are available over the counter.

One of my colleagues recommends "onychial surgery" (picking at warts with the fingernails), but I always worry about the possibility of infection. However, I've never seen a wart get infected, and I suspect that among children an awful lot of onychial surgery goes on that adults don't know about.

Finally, when a wart takes up residence on the sole, or plantar surface, of the foot (plantar warts), they can really be painful. Doughnut-shaped pads made of moleskin or foam rubber will alleviate the pressure on the wart from walking and treat it at the same time. Available at the drugstore, these pads come with self-adhesive. It never works. Add pieces of adhesive tape fore and aft, and the pad will stay on the foot.

If these simple measures fail (or any more exotic ones you'd care to try), you may need your doctor's help. But considering the good prognosis, look for the simplest, least painful, least debilitating, and least expensive treatment available. Good luck.

9

Headaches

The overwhelming majority of all children's headaches originate outside the cranium (the part of the skull that encloses the brain). Brain tissue has no sensory nerve fibers and, therefore, cannot feel pain. Most headache pain is transmitted along blood vessels, either from the face area (eyes, ears, nose, sinuses, upper and lower jaws) or up the back of the neck through the muscles that support the head.

Headache is a symptom rather than a disease. Trying to figure out why a child has a headache involves knowing which conditions are most likely to produce headache and, of these, which one or ones your child is most likely to have. Let's consider the simplest and most obvious causes.

FEBRILE HEADACHES

Toddlers are usually incapable of localizing pain to the head (except in the case of earache), but children four years old or older will often complain of headache during the course of a febrile illness. Frequently the headache will precede the onset of fever by a few hours. This headache is mild and disappears after the first dose of aspirin and usually does not recur even though the fever may wax and wane. No further treatment is necessary unless the headache persists, gets worse, is associated with vomiting or unusual sleepiness. These symptoms require a call to the doctor.

MUSCLE TENSION HEADACHES

I am referring here specifically to the muscle-spasm tension of the back of the head, neck, and shoulders that sets up headache patterns after varying periods of time. The underlying reason for the headache may indeed be emotional, but the actual pain is caused by muscular tension.

Think of the physical tension that builds up in an adult during a long drive at night or in wet weather. Can you feel the ache in your neck and shoulder muscles and the headache that invariably results? Children get this kind of headache, too: after exams or any kind of concentrated activity, in school or out, at any time of day or night.

In addition, any situation that may not be pleasurable for children, even if they're not concentrating, can make them tense, can make their muscles tense, and can therefore set up a headache. This is what I mean by a tension headache.

These headaches may be frequent or recurrent, usually depending on what's really causing them. It is obvious that if a child is unhappy about something on a chronic or long-term basis (for example, a teacher-student problem), this may be the basis for recurrent tension headaches. If another child in the family or a parent gets headaches from time to time, the child is more likely to develop tension headaches. Whether this is a learned experience or an inherited anatomical setup, I don't know; but it has certainly been my experience that tension headaches can run in families.

Tension headaches respond to aspirin and rest. Your child should have his full dosage of aspirin (see Chapter 1). Don't give a smaller dose for a small headache. The full dose will give him more relief, faster, thus cutting down on the necessity for repetitive doses. Encourage him to lie down for a while. Read him a story. But don't let him watch TV—the eyes have to work too hard.

What about prevention, especially in the recurrent cases? What's bugging him? Is he having a problem at school? Perhaps on the school bus? Is there a neighborhood bully? How about extracurricular activities? Are there too many? You can't take his word for this. I've known kids involved in scouting, music lessons, swimming at the Y, religious instruction, varsity sports or intramurals, getting straight A's, and having headaches! Yet they don't want to give anything up. In this situation, you have to be firm.

The more specifically emotional causes of headache may be harder to spot. Many problems upset children, and anything that upsets them can cause headaches. My younger son developed headaches that drove us berserk for two months. (One always thinks of the worst things in doctors' children.) Finally, we worked him up—X rays, eye examination, EEG, the whole bit. Of course we found nothing, and of course, he immediately got better. When we realized that all of the special attention of the work up was what probably cured him, it became clear that he resented his brother's feats on the swim team.

If your child's mood, behavior, and enjoyment of activities are frequently impaired because of headaches, then it's time to seek the doctor's help. He will try to rule out some of the causes I shall describe in the next section, but he will first want to know if there are any emotional situations that may be contributing to the problem. Go through the mental gymnastics beforehand and try to figure out what's bugging the child. Your responses will be more thoroughly thought out, and the doctor will have a better chance of accurately assessing what's behind the headache.

EXTRACRANIAL CAUSES OF HEADACHE

This section will examine other causes of headache, in the head but outside the brain. For all these conditions, you will need your physician's help, but a brief survey can educate you to the possibilities and perhaps point you in the right direction.

Eyes

Visual difficulties may cause headache. The presumed mechanisms are eye strain, eye-muscle tension, and so forth. Farsightedness and astigmatism are the most common causes, with nearsightedness and muscle-balance problems running a close second. Since eye problems are frequently inherited, headaches in school (or while reading) and parents who wear glasses should give you a clue.

Ears

Most ear problems produce ear discomfort, and most children can identify localized ear pain. However, the younger the child and the *less* acute the problem, the more likely he is to respond with irritability and/or headache, rather than with the specific ear complaint.

Nose and Sinuses

Hypoxia (less than enough oxygen in the blood) or hypercapnia (too much carbon dioxide) can cause headaches. It is therefore easy to understand that any condition that interferes with the supply of oxygen to the blood can cause headaches. This includes allergic noses, chronically swollen nasal mucous membranes, chronic sinusitis (which will in time produce chronically swollen nasal mucous membranes), polyps, deviated septa, huge tonsils and adenoids, and even asthma, which forces the child to make an extra effort to breathe. Headaches of this nature often seem to move from the face to the forehead and behind the eyes. They are frequently alleviated by decongestants and/or antihistamines, depending on the problem. Aspirin helps only temporarily; the headaches seem to return almost immediately after the aspirin wears off.

Tooth Pain

Most people who experience tooth pain, either from spontaneous toothache or from a rough experience in the dentist's office, get a headache. But a child with a mild toothache frequently complains about a headache first. Sometimes this starts as face pain, or jaw pain, usually one-sided, which may then spread to the whole side of the head. Obviously, fix the cause and you fix the headache.

THE OTHER 2 PERCENT

This category includes rare causes of headache in children. Diagnosis will certainly depend on your physician, laboratory tests, X rays, or even consultation with a specialist. The chances are good that your child's headache will not be caused by any of these conditions, but you should know about them anyway.

Head Injury

Headache is such a universal symptom in children with head injuries that I'd say any child who bangs his head is entitled to a headache. The headache may or may not be important. What you should look for is what happens to the headache and what the other symptoms are, if any. Vomiting (more than once), sleepiness, unsteadiness of gait, and uncoordinated eye movements are all symptoms that should be brought to your physician's attention. But headache alone deserves watchful waiting.

Migraine

Migraine is a recurrent, severe, one-sided, vascular headache (throbbing, pounding; frequently a blood vessel on the side of the forehead can be seen to pulsate). Most often, it will occur in a child whose family has a history of migraine headaches. It is sometimes accompanied by nausea and vomiting. Your physician should always be consulted if you suspect that migraine may be your child's problem. There are new medications that may ameliorate the course of the headache pattern and even prevent its recurrence.

Other Causes

There are other causes of headache, frequently very serious, that your physician may have to consider in his evaluation of symptoms. Brain tumors, brain abscesses, the congenital malformation of major blood vessels, severe infection, and convulsive disorders are all associated with headache. Obviously, none of these conditions is amenable to home remedies. I mention them only to help you understand the need for X rays, laboratory procedures, consultations, and even hospitalization if they are recommended by your physician. Fortunately, these conditions are all extremely rare.

10

The Eyes and Visual Function

The common eye problems that occur in childhood most often require consultation with your physician or with a specialist. They can, however, usually wait for a routine checkup. Assume this to be the case unless I indicate otherwise.

TURNED EYES (STRABISMUS, OR SQUINT):
REAL AND APPARENT

In the second half of the first year, or shortly thereafter, it is frequently noted that "one of the baby's eyes turns in." This condition is called *strabismus,* or squint. Where squint is real, it represents a true eye muscle problem. But most turned eyes, fortunately, are "optical illusions." Take a look at Figure 17. Notice the prominent fold of skin sweeping out from the bridge of the nose and covering the inner

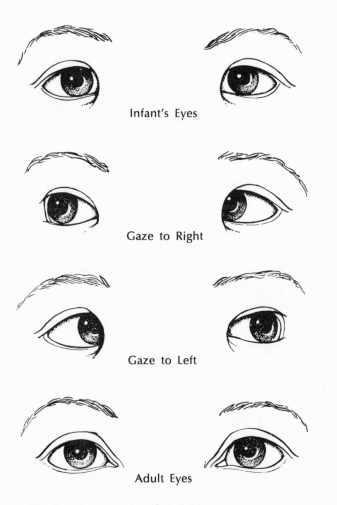

Infant's Eyes

Gaze to Right

Gaze to Left

Adult Eyes

Figure 17. Prominent epicanthal folds may suggest a squint in normal eyes

corner of each eye; many infants have such a fold. When the baby looks to the left, the right eye partially disappears under the fold of skin. Since the observer sees more white to the left of the pupil on the left side, the assumption is made that the right eye turns in too much. The opposite, of course, is apparent when he looks to the right.

Two simple tests will help you to determine whether the squint is more apparent than real. First, try to make the baby look alternately to the left and right. The squint usually will occur equally on both sides. But when the baby has a true eye-muscle problem, the odds are that the squint will occur on only one side. The second test is more sophisticated and may require a little practice. Shine a light at the baby's eyes from a distance of one or two feet so that its reflection appears on the same spot in both eyes. If the baby looks at the light, the reflection should be in the very center of the pupil. If he looks away, it should be in the same spot, relatively, on each eyeball (see Figure 18). If it isn't he may have strabismus. Check with your doctor on the next regular visit.

True squint needs the help of your physician and, usually, an ophthalmologist. Early diagnosis is important in order to prevent blindness. When the eyes don't work together, they cannot fuse their two individual images into one. And since double vision is very uncomfortable, the brain will soon learn to reject or suppress or forget the image of the turned eye, and blindness *may* result.

When the diagnosis of squint is made, the ophthalmologist will frequently try to obstruct vision in the good eye in order to make the child use the weak one. (Turned eyes can be accompanied by other problems, like nearsightedness or astigmatism.) He may obstruct the good eye's vision by patching the eye, by having you administer drops that

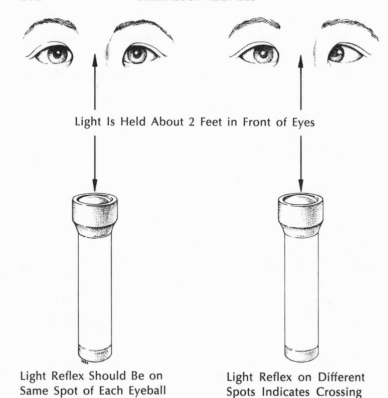

Light Is Held About 2 Feet in Front of Eyes

Light Reflex Should Be on   Light Reflex on Different
Same Spot of Each Eyeball   Spots Indicates Crossing

Figure 18. The flashlight test for squint

will blur the vision temporarily, or even by prescribing
glasses. If these approaches fail, surgery may be required.

INFECTIONS

Infections occur in many areas in and around the eye.
Those inside the eye require the help of a specialist, so you
should always bring a red, angry, painful eye to the atten-

tion of your doctor. You can usually treat the more superficial infections that are discussed here yourself.

Pinkeye (Conjunctivitis)

Pinkeye is an inflammation and/or infection of the conjunctiva, the outermost layer of the white of the eye that extends to become the mucous membrane of the inside of the eyelid. Conjunctivitis may occur as a result of the instillation of silver nitrate in a newborn, as a result of generalized virus infection (see Adeno-Pharyngeal-Conjunctival Fever in Chapter 6), or specifically as an infection of the eyes alone. In the latter instance, it is known popularly as *pinkeye* and appears as reddened eyes, with mucus being produced in varying quantities. The mucus collects in the corners, spills over the lids onto the cheeks, and may even dry on the lashes during the night. The child may awaken terrified because his eyes are stuck shut and he can't open them. Washing them with absorbent cotton and warm water will get them unstuck. A call to your doctor will then be in order.

Antibiotic eye drops are usually prescribed. These will clear the condition quite nicely, although some doctors withhold treatment for a few days in order to give the body a chance to clear the infection by itself. Normal tearing will wash eyedrops out of the eye in twenty minutes, so I usually advise that they be instilled once an hour.

Eye specialists may insist on examining patients with conjunctivitis before ordering treatment. Many pediatricians, however, are willing to treat over the telephone, especially when there are multiple cases in one family (pinkeye can be highly contagious) or when the child has had it before, or when the doctor knows the mother to be a reliable observer. My own feeling is that telephone treatment is often appropriate. But I always examine the child if the conjunctivitis is in only one eye (indicating that a cinder or speck of dirt may be present), or if it does not clear within a day or so with the eyedrops I prescribe.

Red, Scaly Eyelids

This condition, known medically as *chronic blepharitis,* is characterized by red, scaly eyelids and usually is seen in older children. Frequently, one parent has the problem as well. Its cause is unknown, although some doctors believe it occurs more often in allergic families and may therefore be a form of eczema of the eyelids. It doesn't bother the child at all. When treated with ointments, it disappears, but it returns after the treatment is stopped. You're better off leaving red, scaly eyelids alone. They may be with the child for a long time.

Sties

A sty is a pimple or little boil that appears on the edge of the eyelid. There may be more than one sty at a time, and they occur more often in some children than in others. Many doctors prescribe eyelid ointments; I don't because I don't think the medication can get into the sty to do any good. I prefer the old method of hot soaks for boils. The frequent application of moist heat (using a washcloth that has been soaked with hot tap water) for twenty minutes every two hours will usually make the sty either come to a head and drain or disappear without draining.

If hot soaks don't clear the sty within a few days, or

if the sty becomes larger and more tender or painful, your doctor should see it. He should also see children with recurrent sties, for he may be able to discover a focus of infection, or seeding point, and clear the condition once and for all.

Swollen Eyes

"Swollen eyes" is a misnomer—the swelling is actually *around* the eyes. This condition can have a number of causes. The most common cause of swelling of *one* eye is a bug bite, although the child may not know he has been bitten. The area may itch, and the swelling will persist for a few days, always being worse in the morning and getting better as the day progresses. This is due to body position: the head is lower at night and more fluid accumulates. Usually no treatment is necessary.

If the swelling is accompanied by fever and pain, your doctor should be consulted. He will be able to tell whether the source of infection is in the eye, nose, or sinuses. One characteristic of deep sinusitis is the alternate swelling of the eyes, first one and then the other, over a period of several days. It is sometimes mistaken for alternate bug bites.

Swelling around *both* eyes implies increased retention of fluid by the body generally. Unless the child has a history of nasal allergy and upper respiratory obstruction and he is at the height of his allergy season, your physician should see him in order to rule out other, more serious, causes of fluid retention. Incidentally, allergy can actually cause the eyes themselves, and especially the conjunctiva, to swell. In this condition, the conjunctiva will be pale or bluish lavender in appearance, will be quite itchy and uncomfortable, and the child may also have sneezing and nasal obstruction.

VISUAL FUNCTION

Our concern here is with the ability of the eyes to see, to form true and accurate images of the world. Such ability depends on the eye's being constructed in accurate proportions and on the proper functioning of its individual parts. If any one of these conditions is not met, function is impaired. Let's see why defects in visual acuity occur, how they are special in children, and what your doctor can do about them.

Figure 19 shows the similarity so often pointed out between the eye and a camera. An image (composed of light rays) enters the camera (eye) through a filter (cornea) and a shutter (pupil), is concentrated and turned upside down by the lens (lens), and then falls on the film (retina), where an image is made. The brain then interprets the image, turning it right side up in the process, and the eye sees it —in *stereo* (by fusing the images of both eyes) *and* color.

If the proportions of the eyeballs are not perfect, vision is impaired. When the eyeball is too long, the image falls in front of the retina, and the ability of the lens to correct is limited to objects up close. The patient is said to be nearsighted or *myopic*. When the eyeball is too short, the image falls *behind* the retina, and the ability of the lens to correct is limited to objects far away. The patient is said to be *farsighted,* or *hyperopic*.

Sometimes the cornea is improperly curved (like a defect in window glass), and when the patient tries to look through the defect, the shape of the image is distorted. This condition is called *astigmatism*. If the two eyes can't coordinate properly and can't fuse the images, the patient loses *depth perception*. The cause is eye-muscle weakness. And

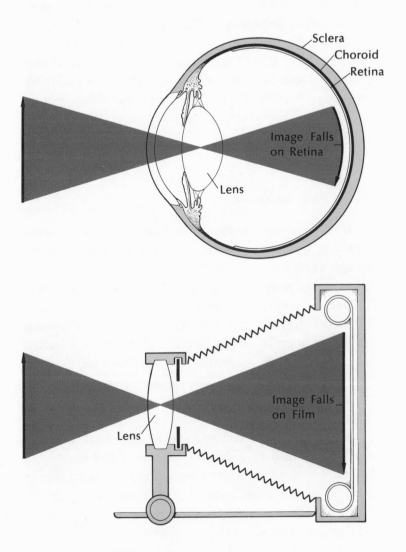

Figure 19. The eye compared to a camera

finally, if the retina lacks certain of the proper receptors for color, the patient is said to be *color-blind*.

Before the visual image can be perceived, assimilated, and understood, it must first be composed, edited, and transmitted. All these functions are accomplished over a complex network of nerve centers in the brain, and things can go wrong in the brain. We are only beginning to understand visual perception problems in children, especially as they relate to learning. More on this below.

Myopia (Nearsightedness)

By far the most common visual acuity problem in children is myopia. The condition is frequently hereditary. Although usually obvious in late childhood and puberty, in severe cases it may be spotted as early as toddlerhood. Toddlers who often *stumble into objects* are suspect. Stumble frequently, not just fall; all toddlers fall. Diagnosis should be actively sought before a child enters school if one or both of his parents is myopic. There are excellent tests for visual acuity that do not require reading skills, and most children can be taught to perform on a vision-testing machine or an eye chart by age four.

When a child is said to have 20/20 vision, it means that he can read at a distance of twenty feet the line of letters he is *supposed* to be able to read at twenty feet in order to be considered normal. If his vision is only 20/70, that means that at twenty feet he reads the line of letters that normal kids can read at seventy feet. This child is myopic, the letters need to be much larger before he can see them. If a child's vision is 20/10, he can see at twenty feet what a normal child would have to be standing at ten feet to see. Supergood? Not really, for this child is probably farsighted and may have trouble seeing things up close.

Childhood eye problems are special because they are so intimately related to growth and development and therefore are extremely important in the early years. We know that newborns perceive light and dark; at three months, they can distinguish shapes and objects; at six months, they can recognize their parents. But it is not until they are five or six years old that they achieve 20/20 visual acuity. (Frequently, four- and five-year-olds can only read 20/30. This is normal.)

In later childhood and prepuberty, children's genetic endowments catch up with them, and they may develop myopia and astigmatism. Within a few years, they can go from 20/20 to 20/200, and there doesn't seem to be a thing that can be done about it except to supplement their natural lenses with eyeglasses.

Hyperopia (Farsightedness)

Farsightedness is rare in children and therefore needs only brief mentioning here. Children with severe hyperopia may test normally for years because their lenses are so supple that they can correct for their anatomical deficit (shortness of the eyeball). But when they get a little older, they will complain of eye strain and headache after long periods of reading.

Astigmatism

Astigmatism is an improper curvature of the cornea (the "window" over the pupil) usually associated with nearsightedness or farsightedness. The diagnosis is made by the eye specialist when he is consulted because the child has a problem in visual acuity. Sometimes it is found as a single defect; it generally produces symptoms of fatigue, eye strain, or headache when the condition is moderately severe.

Eyeglasses

By itself, less than perfect vision in children is no reason for prescribing glasses. Children don't *need* vision that is better than 20/40 or 20/50 to function adequately. When a child starts to squint as he enters the room, when he complains of being unable to see the blackboard from the back of the classroom, when his batting average falls, or he can't catch long fly balls in the outfield, that's the time for him to get his glasses. His appreciation of what they do for him is likely to outweigh his concern for his appearance, which should make the transition a lot easier. Also, an older child is less likely to fall or injure himself while wearing glasses.

There is no point in postponing the prescription of glasses once it becomes necessary. There is no point in discouraging the use of glasses out of fear that the child will come to depend on them or on the assumption that the eyes will learn to work extra hard to become strong. There is no point in forcing bunches of carrots or ounces of cod-liver oil, or large doses of vitamin A on the child in an attempt to strengthen the eyes. Such measures can do more harm than good—particularly excessive doses of vitamins.

As a safety feature, all children's glasses should be made with shatterproof glass. The additional expense may be considered insurance.

THE USE AND ABUSE OF ORTHOPTICS

Orthoptics is a method of visual training, utilizing eye exercises and various lenses, to correct visual defects and improve binocular vision (both eyes working together).

Ophthalmologists are physicians who specialize in diseases of the eye. They are qualified to prescribe and manage the orthoptic training of children. Most ophthalmologists use orthoptics with patients who have eye-muscle imbalances to try to achieve binocular vision. They will frequently try orthoptics before resorting to surgery. Orthoptics are also used after surgery to retrain the eyes to work together.

Optometrists are not physicians. They train in a school of optometry for two years following college to learn to measure visual acuity without the use of drops and to prescribe suitable glasses based on the results of their testing. They are also trained to give eye exercises, with and without lenses, in order to improve a patient's binocular vision and visual acuity.

In the early 1950's, the Gesell Institute of Child Behavior began testing children with *normal* visual acuity who had trouble learning to read, and who seemed to be suffering from disabilities in visual function. Their eyes were anatomically normal, but they couldn't use them properly in reading. A whole school of thought on visual perceptual handicaps emerged, and numerous methods of treatment were devised to help these children. These treatments include countless sessions at orthoptic training, and eyeglasses and other eye devices with severe corrective lenses prescribed for children with anatomically normal visual acuity. It seems to me that proponents of this school, largely optometrists and educators, have very little evidence to support the effectiveness of these methods in the treatment of children's reading problems. Many pediatricians and ophthalmologists view these measures as not only ineffectual but in some cases harmful for most children with normal visual acuity who have reading problems.

All of which suggests that it's a good idea to get several respected opinions (from optometrists, ophthalmologists, and educators, too) before subjecting a child to rigorous orthoptic exercises, with or without lenses, for reading problems.

11

New Advances

PROBLEMS OF GROWTH: TOO TALL AND TOO SHORT

Height is a subject of "quiet" concern to many parents. They don't talk about it in front of the child because they don't want to give him a complex. They may not talk about it with each other because they assume it is inherited. They feel guilty if they think it is inherited from their side of the family, and they don't want to hurt feelings if it's inherited from the other. And they may not want to discuss it with the doctor because it's "too trivial," or he's "too busy," or "everybody knows that nothing can be done about it anyhow." Quiet concern.

Height is usually considered a problem when a boy is too short or a girl is too tall. Occasionally, but infrequently, you hear about a girl being too short, but you almost never hear that a boy is too tall. (Thank basketball for that!) Concern revolves around social discomfort for both boys and girls.

Growth depends on many factors, perhaps the most obvious of which is *heredity*. This factor is one you can't do anything about.

Nutrition, too, is an important factor, since growth depends on it. Poor nutrition produces "runting" (shortness of stature) in experimental animals and turns up as a cause of short stature in some socioeconomic groups. Nutrition also plays a role in the growth of a child *before* birth. Infants of malnourished mothers are shorter than expected and frequently do not achieve their expected potential height regardless of their nutrition after birth.

Hormones, of course, affect height. The pituitary gland produces a growth hormone that is primarily responsible for linear growth and the child's eventual height. Abnormalities in the functioning of this gland can produce extreme shortness of stature or gigantism. The thyroid gland, also, is capable of retarding growth if it functions inadequately.

Finally, unusual *infection,* severe or long-standing, seems to play a role in linear growth, preventing children from reaching their expected height. (Please note that the frequent upper respiratory infections that most children have in the first few years of their lives do not fall into this category. They are a *normal* phenomenon and do *not* retard growth!)

I have referred in the foregoing discussion to "expected" height. This is based on tables of predicted height derived from repeated measurements of large populations of children throughout their growing periods. These tables, of course, are accurate only for average heights of many children in varying age groups, not for individual children. Factors that influence the growth of a child may not be common to a whole population. And since children do not grow at the same rate all the time (they grow more in some years, less in others), a single measure of growth is not so meaningful as a series of measurements taken over a protracted period of time.

Given a series of measurements taken of a child's height through the years, a growth curve may be plotted which will not only describe the *rate* of growth the child has sustained, but also enables you to predict what his rate of growth will be if he continues to grow normally (see growth charts in Appendix 3). This information may be useful in several ways. On the basis of past performance, you can determine whether or not a child is living up to his genetic potential. (By and large, the children of tall parents should be tall and the children of short parents should be short.) In addition, the curve should be observed for any severe deviation from a predicted course. For instance, a child growing in the tall normal range for several years who then shifts over to the short normal or even short *abnormal* range should be evaluated to see if a medical reason (such as inadequate thyroid production) can be found for this change.

Finally, recent medical advances will probably make it possible in the near future to alter height for social or cosmetic reasons. Thus, boys who are "too short" may be given synthetic growth hormone to accelerate their growth so that their eventual height will be greater than predicted. And girls who predict in the six-foot range may be able to have their puberty advanced, thus cutting short the growing years and making them ultimately shorter than predicted. This all may seem unimportant in the context of illness, but it certainly matters to a child who has a height problem.

PIGEON TOES AND FLAT FEET

Feet haven't changed very much over the last fifty years. The same problems of growth and development are with us today. What *has* changed is how these problems are dealt with. Consider footwear, for instance. Do you remember the high sneakers or cleats that professional basketball and football players used to wear? Well, most of them don't any more; they've learned that low shoes are more comfortable and that ankle support really isn't necessary for normal feet. The same is true of baby shoes. I tell young mothers that low sneakers are as good as anything for baby's first walkers. They grip well; they don't impede normal muscle function; they're washable; and they're cheap. Times have changed!

Now let's take a look at the two foot problems most likely to cause parental concern.

Pigeon Toes (Toeing In)

Many children, when they start to walk, toe in with one foot (most often the left) and sometimes with both. If a child toes in, look to the foot, the leg, or the thigh for one or more of three common conditions.

METATARSUS VARUS OR ADDUCTUS. Simply described, in this condition a foot curves inward, from heel to toe, like a big comma (see Figure 20). This usually occurs in both feet, usually appears at birth, can occur in varying degrees, and is easily corrected. It should, however, be diagnosed and treated before the child starts to walk. Severe cases will require plaster casts for a few months; moderate

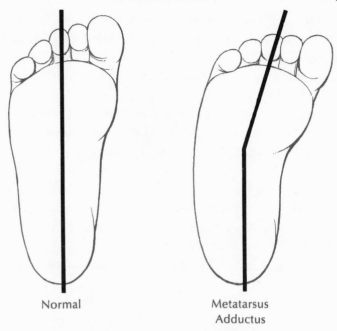

Normal

Metatarsus
Adductus

Figure 20. Metatarsus adductus

cases can be treated with outflare shoes (shoes that flare out at the toes in the opposite direction from the malformity). The simplest cases probably require no correction—that is, they usually correct themselves—but will respond to putting the left shoe on the right foot, and vice versa. This is a simple outflare maneuver. (This, by the way, is the *only* condition that may respond to the reversal of shoes; and even here, it's probably effective only before the child begins to walk.) Most children whose shoes are reversed *after* they start walking will respond with blisters, not correction. Don't do it.

Metatarsus varus is usually caught within the first few months; it does not recur once it has been corrected.

TIBIAL TORSION. In this condition, the tibia, the main bone of the leg, is twisted inward, causing the foot to point in (see Figure 21). It should not be confused with the bowing phenomenon. All babies' legs are bowed at birth and during the first year of life (see Figure 21). This is normal and does *not* rotate the foot inward. Once the baby starts to walk, the stimulation of use will straighten the bow within a very few months. No treatment is necessary.

Tibial torsion is very common. The left leg is more frequently affected (although both legs can be), and the degree of severity varies. The problem is sometimes brought to the physician's attention with the complaint that the opposite leg "points outward too much."

Actually a baby's legs normally assume a froglike posi-

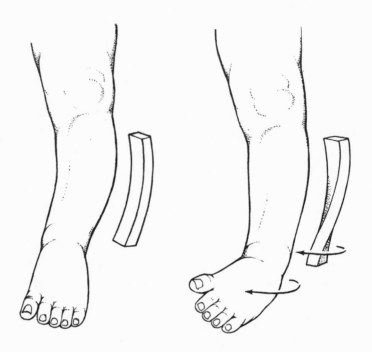

Figure 21. Normal bowing (left) and tibial torsion (right)

tion with each leg rotated outward. But if you bring the knees of a baby with left tibial torsion together, the right foot will usually be straight and the left foot will point inward. And when the baby lies face down on a table or is held against his mother's body (see Figure 22), the feet, instead of pointing outward, point in the same direction (usually to the right if you are looking at the baby from behind). Here again, the right foot is normal; the left points inward. *Internal* tibial torsion is often associated with some degree of metatarsus adductus, which will, of course, make the foot appear to point in even more.

Like the bowing phenomenon, tibial torsion has a remarkable tendency to be self-correcting. However, it has been the experience of many physicians that the correction does not occur spontaneously in all patients. Which conditions do you treat, and which do you leave alone?

The professors say that if you wait long enough, none of them will need correction. They advocate waiting *at least* through the entire first year and then applying corrective devices if necessary. Many doctors, on the other hand, believe this is impractical.

The most popular method of treatment is the *Dennis-Browne Bar;* this is simply a pair of shoes attached to each other by a bar that holds them in a fixed position eight or ten inches apart (see Figure 23). When the infant's feet are in this device, the muscles of his legs continually push against this fixed position. The principle of isometric exercise is utilized to correct the tibial torsion.

I make it a practice to wait until the child is at least five or six months old and consider using the bar only if there has not been significant spontaneous improvement. The key word here is *significant,* since an actual objective measurement of improvement may be difficult to make.

In my experience, the bar has proven to be a safe

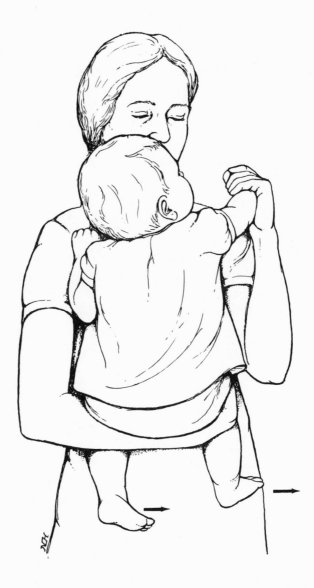

Figure 22. Both feet point the same way

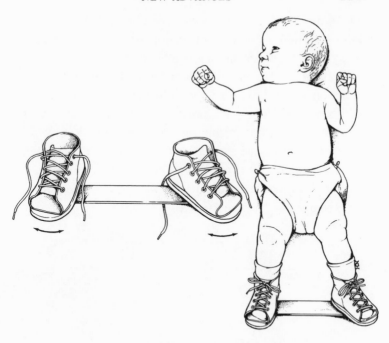

Figure 23. The Dennis-Browne bar

method of treatment and should be used by children whose legs do not significantly straighten by themselves in the first six months of life. The bar is tolerated well in this age group. When used twenty or so hours a day for about three months, I usually find that correction is not only complete but permanent.

FEMORAL TORSION. This cause of toeing in occurs above the knee, in the thigh. The femur (the thigh bone) can be twisted just as the tibia can be twisted inward in tibial torsion. But femoral torsion almost always occurs in both legs. The normal child, with his leg fully extended and the foot pointing straight, can rotate the entire leg about 15 degrees inward and 60 degrees outward (see Figure 24). Examination of a child with femoral torsion will reveal that he is barely able to rotate his legs outward, but he can usually bring them in at almost a 90-degree angle. Have the child lie flat on his back on the floor. If he has this condition, you will see that his foot can be rotated so that the entire inside of his foot, from heel to big toe, can touch the floor.

There are no mechanical devices to correct this condition. Fortunately, it usually straightens out by itself if one is willing to wait long enough. And the waiting game *should* be played—the only alternative is an operative procedure

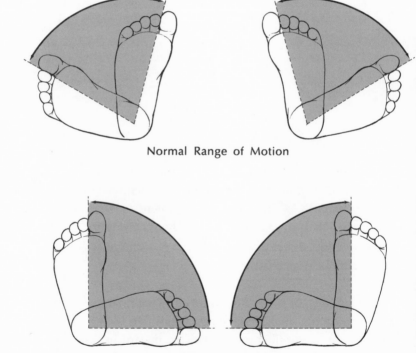

Normal Range of Motion

Femoral Torsion

Figure 24. Rotary motion of legs from the hip

on both legs that requires months of casts and a wheelchair. This massive surgery is almost never indicated.

Flat Feet

All infants and toddlers start out with flat feet. Not actually, but apparently. The question doesn't arise until after he starts to walk. Then it is noted that he does not seem to have an arch. Actually, most children have arches. The arch is obscured by a fat pad that causes the bottom of the foot to look flat. And when the child stands, the inside of his sole appears to touch the ground. His wet footprint will show no arch.

The primary concern in a child with so-called flat feet is not really whether the feet are flat, but rather whether they are pronated (inverted in relation to the ankle). This can best be seen if you look at the standing child from behind. You should be able to draw a straight line from the center of the heel up through the heel cord, *the center of the ankle,* and the center of the knee (see Figure 25). In a child with pronated ankles, a straight line from heel to knee will pass *outside* the ankle joint. This condition requires the help of your physician, who will order corrective devices (arch supports, special shoes, and so forth). In its more severe forms, pronation may be accompanied by knock knees and even toeing *out.* However, these conditions are rare and, should they occur, will certainly be noted by your physician soon after your child starts walking.

One clue to the presence of pronation can be obtained from noting the way a child wears out his shoes. A child with significant pronation will wear the *inside* edge of his soles out as fast as the *inside* edge of the heels. And the

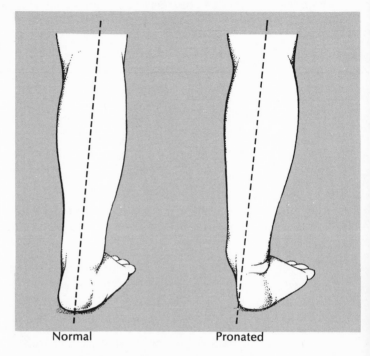

Normal   Pronated

Figure 25. Pronation of the foot

shape of the *inside* of the upper part of the shoe will be broken down as well.

Notwithstanding the possibility of pronation, most children do *not* have flat feet. If your child's legs look straight when you look at him from behind, and if he does not complain of his feet and legs getting tired, the odds are that his feet and legs are in good shape.

PERCEPTUAL HANDICAPS, LEARNING DISORDERS, AND
MINIMAL CEREBRAL DYSFUNCTION

Children may be difficult to raise for one reason or another. Sometimes the difficulty appears early in infancy with the fretful baby, the spitter, or the infant with colic. Sometimes it appears in toddlerhood with temper tantrums (out of all proportion to what one might reasonably expect from a toddler), sleeping problems, or resistance to toilet training. And sometimes difficulties become evident in the preschool and primary-grade years with behavioral disorders arising out of situations at school.

The majority of these problems are variations in the *normal* pattern of growth and development, produced by heredity and environment. Every child, even brothers and sisters living in the same house with the same parents, has an environment different from every other child's. We are never the same parents to each of our children. We're older or younger; we have more or less to do; we're subject to different social and financial pressures; and there are different demands made on us by fewer or more children. And don't forget sibling rivalry. No two children can occupy the same place in the birth order of a family. Even twins have troubles. They are each born slightly different from the other, and parental attitudes, responding to that difference, put them under different pressures.

I dwell on these normal variations to assure you that in most instances where children *have* problems, investigation will usually reveal genetic or environmental factors to explain their "different" behavior. I include in this category all children who are "immature" for their age, first children who are "too good," the middle-child syndrome (whatever that is), the "baby" in the family, and all the other cliché-tagged youngsters one hears about.

However, from this potpourri of possible developmental problems (that is, children whose behavior is not dramatically, but slightly, different), certain categories of children are emerging whose problems may be caused by physical and organic abnormalities. Just as the infant spitter may have a milk allergy and the toddler who gets up at night may have pinworms, so the preschooler may be hyperactive because of minimal cerebral (brain) dysfunction and the third grader may not be able to read because he can't properly fuse the images of both eyes.

Minimal cerebral dysfunction is a term that has come into use in the past few years to describe children with subtle, mild, and limited defects of brain function. It is thought that birth trauma from a difficult delivery, illness during pregnancy, or even a stormy first few days of life may provide the incident that ultimately affects the developing brain. But these factors are often forgotten in the attempt to evaluate the hyperactive toddler whose attention span is virtually nil, whose movements are random and purposeless, and whose only interest seems to be perpetual motion. Lest this description cause too many of you to exclaim, "That's *my* child!" let me assure you that for all the active toddlers seen every day in a pediatrician's office, not ten a year are diagnosed with excessive hyperactivity.

Some children's specific cerebral deficiencies are picked up in the first few years of school. They may have *learning disorders,* problems far more familiar to teachers and special-education people than to a doctor, who deals primarily with physical illness. These specialists can identify children with apparently normal vision who don't see the way you and I do (see "The Use and Abuse of Orthoptics" in Chapter 10 for a discussion of visual perceptual handicaps), or children with apparently normal learning ability who are intelligent but can't comprehend the meaning of certain sounds and may have auditory perceptual handicaps.

Communication disorders occur in children who are intelligent and have normal vocal cords but can't speak in sentences, and in children who can identify printed letters and even words but can't read comprehensively. These also may be examples of minimal cerebral dysfunction.

To further complicate matters, none of these problems occurs in isolated form. The difficulties a child encounters in dealing with his handicap always set up actions and reactions involving the people around him; psychoemotional complications creep in that obscure the diagnosis and invariably affect the treatment. The parents of these children *always* need help in understanding their children's problems, their own reactions to these problems, and the ways in which they can be most supportive in helping their children to overcome or compensate for their handicaps.

Finally, there are certain children whose only manifestation of cerebral dysfunction may be *inordinate clumsiness*. These children may have problems in both major and minor motor skills. They can't do anything well with their bodies. They have trouble running, skipping, heel-and-toe walking, throwing a ball, printing letters, playing with small objects, and doing puzzles requiring simple manual dexterity. They seem to have more than their share of accidents. But these children often do well in school, and after they stop trying to compete with their more athletic peers, they function quite easily in social and classroom situations. Can this really be considered "cerebral dysfunction," or is it more a motor malfunction?

Then again, is this all just semantics? Possibly, but let

me point out that the term you have *not* read here is *brain damage*. Although some of these children have been "damaged" (as opposed to experiencing their ultimate development in any one area), the end result is the same in terms of the current state of medical knowledge. That is, all these children need diagnosis, careful medical and neurological treatment if indicated, and then the most individualized and specialized educational training that can be provided.

ILLNESS BEFORE BIRTH

It has been known for centuries that certain diseases are transmitted from one generation to another. These genetic diseases (caused by defects in the genes) are inherited in varying patterns, depending on the particular genes involved. *Hemophilia,* for instance, is an example of an inherited disorder genetically transmitted by females (who never have the disease) to their male offspring, who bleed excessively.[1]

Not all genetic disorders, however, come down through long lines of inheritance. Sometimes only an occasional gene in a man or woman's chromosomal makeup will be abnormal, so that a defective offspring shows up only sporadically, as in congenital heart disease.

More recently, scientists have learned that events occur-

1. Although hemophilia was first described clinically in the 1740's, there is evidence that the Jews had a basic understanding of the hereditary mechanism a thousand years earlier. In the Talmud they instructed that if a woman bore two sons consecutively who died of weakness (bleeding at circumcision), the third son should not be circumcized until he was an adult. Further, if a sister of the unfortunate woman bore a son (even her first), he also was not to be circumsized until later.

ring *during* pregnancy can have an adverse effect on the fetus. Certain drugs (thalidomide, for instance), infection (such as rubella), and radiation have all been incriminated. Maternal smoking has been associated with low birth weight, and poor nutrition is a setup for "runting," or babies with low birth weight.

Most inherited genetic disorders were shrugged off as unfortunate medical curiosities until recently. But during the last few years, a combination of events has made it possible to *do* something about some of them.

Rh Disease

The saga of the *Rh problem* contains elements of nearly all these recent advances; it provided the impetus for much of the research in the field and is probably the commonest condition seen in the hereditary-genetic spectrum.

The Rh factor is a substance found in the red blood cells of 85 percent of the population. These people are designated as *Rh positive*. The remaining 15 percent of the population, who lack the factor, are called *Rh negative*. If an Rh negative woman carries an Rh positive fetus, the father has to be Rh positive. (See Appendix 4 for a diagram outlining the genetic possibilities for offspring of Rh negative mothers.)

When an Rh negative woman carries an Rh positive fetus, small quantities of the baby's Rh positive blood may cross the placenta and enter the mother's bloodstream. The Rh factor can "sensitize" the mother and cause her to produce antibodies against that factor, much as we sensitize or immunize a person against tetanus by injecting tetanus protein. These maternal antibodies are then capable of crossing the placenta and going into the fetus's bloodstream, where they attack and destroy red blood cells which carry the Rh factor.

Consequently, Rh diseased babies can be born anemic or can get into trouble shortly after birth because they become severely jaundiced. Doctors have learned to treat this kind of jaundice by changing the baby's blood in the first day or two of life. Using Rh negative blood, by means of an *exchange transfusion,* most of the bilirubin (the breakdown product of blood that causes jaundice) and antibodies can be washed out. Since the baby is being given Rh negative blood, there are very few Rh positive red blood cells on which remaining antibodies can act. In the four months following this exchange, the infant will replace the transfused negative blood with his own positive blood; but by this time, there will be too few antibodies left to do any damage.

Recently, phototherapy, a form of light treatment, has been used to hasten the breakdown of bilirubin into nontoxic products that are more readily excreted by the infant. The figures are not in yet, but I believe they will show that phototherapy can reduce the necessity of exchange transfusion significantly.

A special *Rh gamma globulin* has been developed that virtually stops the production of antibodies when injected into Rh negative mothers of Rh positive newborns within a day or two after delivery. Thus, each subsequent pregnancy "acts like" a first pregnancy, and the newborn is not afflicted with Rh disease.

Amniocentesis

Amniocentesis is a relatively new technique which enables a doctor to know more about the condition of an unborn baby than has ever been possible before. Through testing a specimen of the amniotic fluid (the liquid in the bag of waters surrounding the baby) in various ways, it has become possible to determine how severely a baby is affected by Rh disease, and to treat the baby with intrauterine transfusions (yes, even this is possible now) or even to deliver the baby early, thus stopping his exposure to maternal antibodies.

Similarly, in women with known genetic disorders, which are transmissible, examining the chromosomes of cells floating around in the amniotic fluid can reveal the sex of the baby and *may* reveal whether or not the fetus is a victim of the disease in question.

Interruption of Pregnancy

In the absence of the ability of medicine to treat such conditions, the liberalization of abortion laws in many states gives parents new prerogatives in the determination of their offspring. A woman who knows she is a hemophilia carrier, for instance, can undergo amniocentesis and find out whether her baby is a boy or girl. A girl will not have hemophilia (although she may be a carrier); a boy is likely to be a bleeder. Many states will allow the mother the choice of keeping or aborting the fetus. Similarly, some women are more likely to produce mongoloid babies. Here again, amniocentesis and examination of recovered cells and chromosomes can provide her with the answer to the ever-present question, "Doctor, will my baby be normal?" If the answer is no, the parents may wish to have their defective offspring aborted.

Obviously, this all raises many legal, moral, and religious issues that need to be considered very carefully by parents and doctor. It is my own feeling that the health and well-being of parents and children should be the paramount concern.

One final thought: In this Huxleyan world we are entering, one aspect of the doctor-patient relationship will be reversed. Time was when the patient always gave the doctor the symptoms and the doctor told the patient what to do. Now, in certain situations, the doctor (geneticist) can give the patient certain genetic facts and hard statistical probabilities, but the patient has to make the final judgment. And this is as it should be.

The future promises even more amazing possibilities. With specific genetic diagnosis becoming more of a reality, treatment may be just over the horizon. Screening for defective babies, selection of cells for reproduction, even specific selection of genes, may be feasible. Hopefully, these discoveries will eventually enable us to prevent genetic defects and accidents of nature. Who knows? By then the world may even be a better place for those better human beings we create to live in it.

PART II

Glossary

This is a glossary of additional diseases, conditions, and other terms, arranged alphabetically for ready reference.

ABO incompatibility. A woman who is blood type O has no type A or type B substance in her blood. An infant who is type A has A substance; an infant who is type B has B substance. Just as in Rh disease, it is possible, if an infant has type A or type B blood, for some of that blood to pass into the mother's bloodstream. She may then produce antibodies to A or B substance and pass them back to the infant, thereby destroying some of the infant's blood. Erythroblastosis fetalis (which see) may occur in the infant so affected.

Generally speaking, erythroblastosis that results from ABO incompatibility is less severe than Rh disease, but the symptoms and treatment are generally the same. For a further discussion of the mechanism see page 229.

Abscess. A localized area of infection in and under the skin, the central portion of which has become liquefied. An abscess almost invariably needs to drain or be drained. This may be hastened by the application of warm soaks as frequently as possible. They should be continued through the drainage process until the infection becomes quiescent. Fever accompanying the abscess means that the infection may have spread beyond the localized area, and a physician should be consulted. See page 186.

Acid. A slang expression for LSD, an hallucinogenic drug.

Acidosis. An imbalance of the normal acid-alkaline ratio of the blood toward the acid side. This condition is commonly seen in gastroenteritis when vomiting and diarrhea are severe. For a discussion of the diagnosis and treatment of dehydration, which usually precedes acidosis, see page 120.

Acne. Excessive oiliness of the skin which leads to blemishes, pimples, and blackheads, most commonly seen in adolescents. See page 187.

Achromycin. A broad-spectrum antibiotic. The generic name is tetracycline. It is not used very much any more in small children because of the possibility of permanent staining of the teeth. However, it is used frequently in teen-agers for primary atypical pneumonia and bronchitis and sometimes in the treatment of acne.

Adenitis. An inflammation and enlargement of lymph glands, usually associated with infection. The affected glands will be localized when the infection is a local one (e.g., swollen neck glands with sore throat). Or the lymph glands may be generally swollen all over the body, which frequently occurs in viral infections like infectious mononucleosis. See page 87.

Adenoids. Lymphatic tissue located in the front and the back of the nasal portion of the throat. Notorious for their ability to cause mouth breathing, snoring, and obstruction of the opening of the eustachian tube going out to the ear, thereby producing middle-ear infection. See page 85.

Adenovirus. An upper respiratory virus which commonly swells lymph glands in the area of the throat and neck. See page 160.

Adrenalin. A hormone secreted by the adrenal glands. Used as a medication given by injection in the treatment of severe allergic reactions and shock.

Airsickness. A form of motion sickness generally associated with riding in an airplane. However, children frequently experience airsickness from carnival rides. See Appendix 2.

Albumin in urine. Commonly associated with disease of the kidneys. Adolescents frequently have albumin in the urine in small amounts. This is of no consequence.

Alopecia. Hair loss occurring in small round areas of the scalp. The cause of this condition is unknown; treatment is not usually necessary, and hair returns, generally within a few months.

Amblyopia. A lessening of vision, usually in one eye, sometimes without obvious cause. This condition is frequently seen in children with a turned eye. When two eyes are incapable of focusing on one object, double vision occurs. Since double vision is very uncomfortable to the child, he may suppress the vision in the turned eye, resulting in amblyopia. See discussion of strabismus, page 199.

Ammonia dermatitis. A redness, or "scalding," of the skin caused by urine that contains an unusually large quantity of an ammonia salt. This changes to ammonia on standing. See page 173.

Amniocentesis. The sampling of the amniotic fluid (the bag of waters surrounding the baby) before birth, in order to examine it. Much can be learned, including blood type, Rh factor, sex, and the presence of Rh disease. This procedure is not performed casually—it is done only when it becomes important to obtain specific information. See page 231.

Amphetamines. Stimulant drugs, or "uppers."

Ampicillin. A form of penicillin which has a much broader spectrum of action than regular penicillin. This antibiotic is frequently used in infants and younger children whose bacterial infection may be different from the type of infection seen in older children. It frequently causes diarrhea, which is a side effect, not an allergic reaction.

Anemia. Inadequate blood. There are many types, The commonest in children is iron-deficiency anemia, frequently seen in infants in the first year of life and in toddlers.

Animal bites. There are three areas of primary concern in animal bites. The first, local infection, should be treated with adequate cleansing and scrubbing. The second, the possibility of tetanus infection, will be handled by adequate immunization (see Appendix 1). The third, the possibility of rabies, is virtually nonexistent in controlled pets and domestic animals. In the case of an animal bite of a wild animal or an unknown pet, your physician should be consulted.

Anorexia. Extreme loss of appetite. It is commonly seen in certain nervous disorders, most especially of the female adolescent (anorexia nervosa). Some diseases, such as hepatitis, cause mild anorexia.

Antibiotic. A type of medication specifically designed to fight bacterial infection. For a discussion of the effect of antibiotics as they relate to bacterial as opposed to viral infections, see page 36.

Antidotes. Medicines used to counteract the effects of poisons, usually taken internally. See the discussion of accidental poisoning on page 48.

Antifungal medicine. If local or topical medication does not alleviate the problem, it is possible to use internal medication,

which is sometimes more effective. Your physician must prescribe these drugs. See Appendix 2.

Antihistamines. Medicines designed to counteract the effect of
histamines, i.e., natural substances released in excessive quantities in allergic reactions. See Chapter 5 and Appendix 2.

Antipyretics. Medicines designed to bring down fever. See the
discussion on aspirin, page 45, and Appendix 2.

Aphasia. The loss or impairment of the ability to use words as
symbols of ideas.

Arthritis. Commonly considered a disease of old age, arthritis
may occur in children. A rare form of juvenile rheumatoid arthritis exists, and mild arthritis is seen as a complication of
many common childhood illnesses.

Ascorbic acid. Commonly known as vitamin C, this drug has
achieved recent fame (or notoriety) in its alleged ability to ward
off a common cold. This ability has never been proven by accepted medical studies. In addition, the toxicity of some recommended high doses of ascorbic acid when given to children has
never been determined. I cannot recommend the use of ascorbic
acid in doses that exceed 250 milligrams per day in toddlers,
500 milligrams per day in older children, and 1,000 milligrams
per day in adults.

Asian flu. A common and simple upper respiratory infection,
due to a virus and appearing in winter epidemics from time
to time. The term "Asian" is derived from its first isolation in
Hong Kong and has no implication of severity. See the discussion of viral upper respiratory infections on page 62.

Athlete's foot. A localized fungus infection occurring between
the toes, most often in the summertime. For treatment, see Appendix 2. Also see the differential diagnosis of athlete's foot and
eczema on page 183.

Atopic dermatitis. A synonym for eczema.

Aura of epilepsy. An anticipatory feeling, generally lasting seconds or minutes, prior to the onset of a convulsion.

Autism. A form of psychosis seen in children generally under two years of age and categorized as a form of infantile schizophrenia.

Bacitracin. An antibiotic commonly used in local preparations rather than taken internally. It is usually found in antibiotic ointments.

Bag of waters. See Amniocentesis.

Bald spots. See Alopecia.

Barbiturates. ("downers") A drug commonly used for sedation. However, barbiturates, instead of sedating, seem to stimulate some children.

Battered child syndrome. A complex of traumatic injuries (including broken bones) seen in children who have been illegally beaten by adults.

BCG. A vaccine used to temporarily protect an individual against tuberculosis. It is not commonly dispensed in the United States unless there is unusually high risk of exposure to tuberculosis.

Bed wetting. Most often a psychological symptom of delayed development, bed wetting sometimes indicates the presence of urinary-tract infection. See page 128.

Bee stings. Your child is *not* allergic to bee (or wasp, hornet, yellow jacket) stings unless he has hives all over, has difficulty breathing (he feels that his throat is closing up), or is wheezing. If one of these symptoms is present, he should be seen by a physician quickly. If this is not the case, refer to page 149.

Belladonna, Tincture of. A medication used to slow the action of the stomach and the intestines.

Benadryl. An antihistamine commonly used in allergic conditions, but also remarkable for its mild sedative and tranquilizing qualities.

Birth injuries. Injuries that may occur to the newborn infant as a result of the physical trauma suffered during a difficult delivery. See page 226.

Birthmarks. Areas of abnormal pigmentation of the skin noted at or shortly after birth. See page 171.

Blackheads. Pimples with black centers, commonly seen in acne, and representing the accumulation of minute particles of dirt which obstruct the opening of sweat or oil glands. See "Acne" in Chapter 8.

Blepharitis. Redness or scaliness of the eyelids, commonly seen in children with very dry skin and in some allergic children. This condition can be treated and alleviated, but as soon as the treatment is discontinued, it usually returns. Since it does not usually affect the performance of the child (although it doesn't look very nice), my advice is to leave it alone. See page 204.

Blood poisoning. Generally, the spread of an infection from a localized area somewhere on the body, through the lymphatics and into the blood stream. When this occurs, lymphatic glands adjacent to the originally infected area usually get swollen, and the patient develops generalized symptoms of fever and illness. Your physician should be consulted.

Blue baby. A baby with congenital heart disease whose blood is not being adequately supplied with oxygen. This condition is called cyanosis.

Breast pump. A device for pumping the milk out of the breasts of lactating mothers. It may be used to keep the milk supply coming from a mother who is separated from her child, or in certain instances to help the mother whose nipples have become cracked and irritated and need a rest from a vigorously sucking infant.

Breath-holding spells. A phenomenon that occurs in older infants and small toddlers when they begin to cry and hold the first phase of breathing out. This almost always occurs after the first vocal sound. The infant may hold his breath for so long that his color turns dusky blue, and he may actually pass out. I have never known an infant to die or be seriously damaged by a breath-holding spell. Invariably they start breathing again and, if they have become unconscious, return to normal within a few seconds or a minute or so. The spells have no permanent aftereffects and therefore should be no cause for concern.

Breech delivery. The delivery of an infant buttocks-first instead of the usual head-first.

Cancer. A large category of diseases characterized by malignant overgrowth of a tumor, organ, or cell type within the body. In the present state of our knowledge most cancers end fatally. Children as well as adults develop cancer. The commonest kinds of cancer in children are cancer of the white blood cells, or leukemia, and cancers of the eye and the abdomen.

Canker sores. A white ulcerlike sore of the mucous membrane of the mouth caused by a virus. No good treatment is known; the patients invariably get well by themselves. During their presence, spicy, citrus, or salty foods are not appreciated!

Carbuncle. A form of abscess in which there may be multiple cores or openings through which pus can drain.

Cardiac murmur. See Heart murmur.

Cardiovascular collapse. Shock or inadequate blood pressure. Although most commonly seen in instances of blood loss, as in a child who is bleeding from a wound or internally, it can also be seen in a child who loses excessive amounts of fluids from vomiting and diarrhea, with consequent dehydration. The symptoms of shock are paleness, sweating, upset stomach, and lassitude progressing to drowsiness. These symptoms, in a child who has suffered dehydration, should precipitate an urgent call to your physician.

Carotene. A yellow or orange pigment found in carrots, squash, sweet potatoes, and yams. When infants are fed goodly quantities of these vegetables, their skin may take on a yellow cast. This is harmless and is outgrown.

Carsickness. A form of motion sickness characterized by nausea and vomiting occurring when a person rides in an automobile. See Appendix 2 for medication to treat or prevent motion sickness.

Cascara. A mild laxative.

Castor oil. A laxative.

Cat-scratch disease. Enlargement and swelling of a lymph node which drains an area of skin that has been scratched by a cat. Since the lymph node or gland will not enlarge and swell until several days after the initial cat scratch, the scratch itself may be forgotten, and the patient is seen because of presumed primary enlargement and swelling of the gland. Since the lymph gland may need to be drained, and since secondary bacterial infection may have to be treated with antibiotics, a physician should be consulted.

Catarrh, vernal. Redness of the whites of the eyes seen in allergic children in the spring, summer, and fall. No treatment is required unless the eyes are irritated or itchy. If this occurs, your physician should be consulted; he may prescribe soothing eyedrops.

Cathartics. Laxatives. See Appendix 2.

Cauterize. To apply a chemical to stop bleeding or destroy tissue. This may also be done with electricity.

Cavities, dental. Although this condition never killed anyone, it is so widespread in our population that it deserves mention here. Dental cavities can and should be prevented by regular visits to the dentist, the fluoridation of water supplies, the administration of fluoride to the diet of children who do not drink fluoridated water, and good dental hygiene.

Celiac disease. An old name for a condition that is probably food intolerance in varying degrees and to varying foods in infants and toddlers. Currently, in most situations the term generally implies food intolerance to wheat and wheat products.

Cephalhematoma. A localized swelling on the head of a newborn. The swelling is made up of a collection of blood outside the skull and either under the skin or between the bony plate of the skull and one of its fibrous linings. Cephalhematomas always disappear spontaneously, require no treatment, and have a good prognosis. By themselves, they do *not* cause brain damage or any other serious malady of the newborn.

Cerebral palsy. Weakness or paralysis of one or more limbs as a result of damage to the nervous system before or during birth. Actually, this is a very nonspecific diagnosis; the term should probably be abandoned.

Cerumen. Earwax. If a child develops large accumulations of earwax which continually drain from the ear or impede the inspection of the eardrum, your physician may prescribe special ear drops to dissolve and liquefy the wax. Debrox is one such preparation. It may be instilled in the ears once or twice a day for a week and will usually cause the wax to liquefy and drain satisfactorily.

Cesarean section. An operation for the removal of an infant from his mother's womb through her abdomen if vaginal delivery is not possible.

Charley horse. A sore muscle which has been exercised too severely.

Checkup. A routine, periodic physical examination. Checkups are usually done between five and twelve times in the first year of life, between two and four times in the second year, and then with diminishing frequency until the age of three to five, when they are recommended yearly.

Chest X ray. A radiographic picture of the chest and its contents. In children chest X rays are most frequently used to examine for size and configuration of the heart or for evidence of tuberculosis or pneumonia. In the examination for tuberculosis, chest X rays are not usually taken unless the tuberculin tine test is positive. See Appendix 1.

Chiropodist. A person, not a physician, who has special training in the care of foot ailments. Sometimes called a podiatrist, he is usually licensed to practice only his specialty.

Chiropractor. A person who attempts to treat various ailments by manipulation of the skeletal system. The theory of chiropractic is that many ailments occur as a result of abnormalities of the spinal column. Chiropractors therefore manipulate bones (most especially the spinal column) in an attempt to alleviate these ailments. Chiropractors are not physicians. In my opinion chiropractic is dangerous.

Chloromycetin. A brand name for a very special antibiotic. It is not commonly used for children.

Chlor-Trimeton. A brand name for an antihistamine.

Choking. In children, this usually means misplaced food or a foreign object in the windpipe or trachea, rather than in the stomach. A good treatment for choking infants and small children is to hold them upside down and pound them on the back. Larger children will usually bend over themselves as they cough and try to eliminate the misplaced food or object. If there is a possibility that the food or object is of an oily nature (peanuts or oily liquid), it is best to consult your physician.

Cholera. A gastrointestinal infection manifested by severe diarrhea. Fortunately, there is very little cholera in the United States; for foreign travel immunization is available.

Chorea. A manifestation of acute rheumatic fever characterized by involuntary movements of the extremities, head, and tongue. Fortunately, this condition is very rare. Also called St. Vitus's dance.

Chromosome. A strand of protein in the nucleus of a cell which contains genes, or determinants of hereditary characteristics.

Circumcision. An operation, usually performed at birth, for removal of the foreskin of the penis. For a discussion of the pros and cons of circumcision, see page 169.

Cleft palate. A congenital abnormality in which some portion of the roof of the mouth fails to form completely. This condition will be diagnosed by your physician at birth.

Clubfoot. A congenital abnormality of the foot, which will be diagnosed by your physician at birth.

Cod liver oil. A preparation used to supply vitamins A and D to the infant. This has largely been supplanted by more purified vitamins. However, currently it is used in a number of bland ointments which may be recommended for diaper rash.

Codeine. A narcotic drug whose main functions are the alleviation of pain and the treatment of hacking irritative cough. It requires a prescription.

Cold. A simple viral upper respiratory infection characterized by runny nose, hacking cough, irritated throat, low-grade fever, and a feeling of not being well. See page 62.

Colic. Abdominal discomfort in infants, most commonly seen in the second and third months of life. Colic is apt to occur at the same time every day and last for varying periods. One must assure oneself that the baby is clean, dry, well-fed, and well-burped. Treatments include walking the baby; putting a pacifier in his mouth; feeding him a little warm water, a quarter of a teaspoon of paregoric in a little water or fruit juice, or half a teaspoon of your favorite liqueur; applying a warm (not hot) water bottle to his abdomen; increased efforts at burping; and finally, putting him in his crib, closing the door, and turning up the radio. Be assured that he will outgrow colic in a month or so, although until he does, it may be difficult to bear for both parents and child.

Colitis, ulcerative. A chronically inflamed colon seen in adolescents, especially females, causing diarrhea, sometimes bloody, over prolonged periods of time. Symptoms such as this should be brought to the attention of your physician.

Color blindness. Inability to see certain colors. This condition is frequently hereditary, it never changes, and there is no cure.

Colostrum. A thick secretion of the breast, resembling cream, which appears just before milk starts to flow. Colostrum is loaded with antibodies and is beneficial to the newborn infant.

Coma. A state of profound unconsciousness which can occur as a result of head injury or in certain diseases. When you think your child is in a coma, your physician should be summoned immediately.

Concussion. Any injury to the head that results in symptoms other than local pain. Such symptoms may be generalized headache, dizziness, nausea, unsteadiness of gait, or even convulsions. If any of these symptoms appear, consult your physician.

Congenital heart disease. Improper function of the heart as a consequence of abnormal anatomy present from birth. Congenital heart disease will usually be diagnosed by your child's physician in one of his checkups.

Conjunctivitis. Inflammation or infection of the mucous membrane of the eye. See page 203.

Constipation. Abnormally hard, dry infrequent bowel movements. See page 122 and Appendix 2.

Consumption. An old lay expression for tuberculosis. See Appendix 1 for a regimen of diagnostic prevention of tuberculosis utilizing the tuberculin tine test.

Contact dermatitis. Skin rash occurring as a result of the skin touching a substance to which it has become allergic. The commonest example is poison ivy.

Convulsions. Involuntary muscular spasms of one muscle or several sets of muscles due to abnormal nerve impulses which emanate from the brain. There are many different types of convulsions seen in children, the commonest being febrile convulsions. See page 37.

Coombs' test. A blood test used in children, primarily in the newborn, to ascertain whether or not Rh disease or ABO incompatibility is present.

Cord, umbilical. The structure that extends between the infant and the maternal placenta to supply the fetus with nutrients and oxygen during his life in the uterus.

Cornea. The "window" of the eyeball. See page 207.

Cortisone. A medication simulating the action of a hormone of the adrenal gland. It has many uses in many conditions.

Cough. See page 89. See also Appendix 2.

Cough medicines. See Appendix 2.

Crab lice. A species of louse that inhabits pubic hair rather than body hair or hair on the head. In children, since there are generally no pubic hairs, the louse is apt to inhabit eyelashes or eyebrows.

Cradle cap. A scaliness of the head of infants, sometimes related to seborrhea (a skin condition), but more often due to lack of stimulation of the scalp because of maternal fear of injuring the head when shampooing. The condition is usually readily treated with vigorous massage during head washings. Oil may help loosen the scales.

Cramps. See Chapter 4, "Bellyache."

Cretinism. A lay expression for hypothyroidism in infants and small children.

Crib death. Unexplained death occurring in young infants, usually two to four months old, and more frequently in boys than girls. Most often, the cause of death is not found, even at autopsy, although occasionally overwhelming infection or congenital abnormality is discovered. Fortunately, this is a rare occurrence. It is completely unpredictable.

Curvature of the spine. An abnormal configuration of the spine which occurs mostly in girls, usually in the second decade of life. The abnormal curve is usually in the chest and lower back area and goes from left to right or right to left rather than from front to back. This type of curvature is called scoliosis or kyphoscoliosis.

Cyanosis. A bluish discoloration of the skin, usually due to inadequate oxygenation of blood. It is commonly seen in certain types of congenital heart disease.

Cystic fibrosis of the pancreas. A generalized hereditary disease of many mucus-secreting glands of the body. The mucus is too thick to be adequately excreted. Most commonly affecting the lungs and pancreas, it is a grave disease and eventually fatal, but fortunately, it is quite rare.

Cystitis. Inflammation of the urinary bladder. Although other cystic structures of the body may be inflamed and therefore carry the connotation of cystitis, in children it generally refers to the urinary bladder.

Dandruff. A scaly or flaky condition of the scalp, usually seen in older children. Commonly treated with varying forms of medicated shampoo, it is not a serious condition.

Decongestant. A medication given by mouth which helps to dry mucous membranes when children have colds and upper respiratory infections. For varying types of decongestants, see Appendix 2.

Dehydration. Loss of body fluids associated with vomiting and diarrhea. See page 120.

Dental caries. See Cavities, dental.

Dermatitis. An inflammation, infection, or other condition of the skin.

Dermatographia. Small amounts of pressure brought against the skin cause it to react in an allergic fashion by producing a white elevation surrounded by an area of redness. These are called wheals and flares and frequently look like hives or allergic manifestations; they disappear within a few moments. This condition is not serious as far as we know.

Dermatologist. A physician who specializes in diseases of the skin.

Desenex. A drug applied locally to treat superficial fungus infections of the skin such as athlete's foot.

Desensitization. The process of administering small amounts of an allergen over prolonged periods of time in an effort to diminish a patient's allergic reaction to that allergen.

Dexedrene. A stimulant medication.

Dextrose. A simple form of sugar sometimes added to infants' formulas to increase the caloric content.

Diabetes. In its commonest form, a metabolic disease characterized by an inadequate supply of insulin, one of the hormones excreted by the pancreas gland. As a result of this condition, the patient develops symptoms secondary to an elevated blood sugar, the commonest of which are increased eating and drinking and excessive urination.

Dialysis. The process of washing an undesirable chemical out of the bloodstream. Dialysis may be performed directly on the blood, or it may be performed by instilling solutions into the peritoneal cavity and then removing them.

Dick test. A test used to determine susceptibility to scarlet fever. This test is not used very much any more.

Digitalis. A medication used to strengthen the action of the heart.

Dilantin. A medication used to diminish the frequency of certain kinds of convulsions. This is a brand name for a drug whose generic name is diphenylhydantoin. Many new uses have recently been advocated for this drug. It is used in certain types of pulse irregularity and in some migraine headaches in children; it has also been advocated for certain behavioral problems. Good results on these latter uses remain to be published.

Diphtheria. A bacterial infection, predominantly of the throat, which has almost disappeared from the United States as the result of immunization. See Appendix 1.

Diplopia. Seeing double, or seeing two images at the same time.

Diuretics. Drugs that increase the amount of urination and therefore get rid of excess body fluid.

Divergent strabismus. This expression usually refers to weak outer muscles in one or both eyes, such that when one eye looks straight the other seems to look out. Sometimes called "wall-eyed." See page 199.

Down's syndrome. Another name for mongolism.

DPT. The abbreviation for the vaccine to immunize infants against diphtheria, pertussis (whooping cough), and tetanus. See Appendix 1.

Dramamine. A drug commonly used to alleviate or prevent the symptoms of motion sickness.

Drooling. Excessive saliva which intermittently flows out of the mouth. It is commonly associated with teething in infants and small children.

DT. The vaccine used to continue the immunization against diphtheria and tetanus. The vaccination is commonly called a booster shot. See Appendix 1.

Dysentery. Diarrhea of an infectious nature, frequently severe and accompanied by blood and mucus.

Earache. This may have a number of causes, not all of which are an emergency. Earaches can be treated with aspirin and codeine if this has been previously prescribed. If it has not, it may be helpful to give the child some cough medicine that contains codeine. Good doses are a teaspoonful for a one- to three-year-old and two teaspoonsful for the three- to eight-year-old. Above the age of eight, two or three teaspoonsful may be necessary. See pages 68 and 75.

Electrocardiogram (ECG or EKG). A tracing of the electrical impulses of the heart; a diagnostic tool for diagnosing certain types of heart disease.

Electroencephalogram. A tracing of the electrical impulses from the brain; a diagnostic tool which is useful in diagnosing certain abnormalities of the brain, such as epilepsy.

Electrolytes. Certain chemicals in the blood whose values become abnormal as a result of dehydration and fluid imbalance. They are usually corrected by giving intravenous solutions containing electrolyte chemicals.

Emetic. Medication given to make a child vomit. In cases of poisoning or suspected poisoning, the best emetic to use is syrup of ipecac (not "ipecac fluid extract"). This can be given to any child in a dose of one tablespoonful and repeated in thirty minutes if the child does not vomit. It should not, however, be given in cases of suspected poisoning with caustic agents such as lye or Drano or with volatile chemicals like gasoline, kerosene, and cleaning fluid.

Encephalitis. An inflammation of the brain, generally caused by a viral or bacterial infection. Encephalitis is much more common than was previously supposed. Mild encephalitis may occur with diseases as simple as chicken pox and mumps. It may also be a frequent finding in otherwise ordinary nonspecific virus diseases. The commonest symptoms are high fever, headache, nausea, vomiting, and excessive sleepiness. Your physician should be consulted if encephalitis is suspected.

Encephalogram. See Electroencephalogram.

Endocrine glands. Glands that secrete hormones directly into the bloodstream. Examples are the pituitary, thyroid, and adrenal glands.

Enema. The introduction of fluid into the rectum. Enemas may be given to help a child have a bowel movement, sometimes even as a method of giving a child fluids. *Caution*: Large volumes of pure water or soap suds should not be given to small children. It is possible to wash out certain chemicals in the body and throw them into electrolytic imbalance.

Enteritis. An inflammation of the intestinal tract, usually the small intestine. The symptoms are vomiting and diarrhea.

Enuresis. Bed wetting. The term usually refers to nocturnal enuresis, or night-time bed wetting. Bakwin has studied this problem at great length and finds that there is a parental history of bed wetting in 75 to 80 percent of cases. Most authors do not consider that a problem exists until the age of five or six years. Treatment has gone through phases of water restriction (to lighten the load), water excess (to stretch the bladder and increase capacity), medicine to tighten the outflow valve of the bladder, medicine to loosen the outflow valve of the bladder, etc.

The current state of the art is to administer tranquilizers at bedtime. These children seem to sleep very soundly; it is thought that they have burrowed very deeply into their subconscious mind and wet the bed as they did in infancy. Tranquilizers seem to make them sleep *less* soundly, and thus the child does not perform in an infantile fashion. In addition, if he really does have a full bladder, he can get up more easily.

For a small number of children with recurrent urinary-tract infection, nocturnal enuresis may herald the onset of another infection. Urinalysis or urine culture may be indicated.

Eosinophiles. A kind of white blood cell (leucocyte) found in the blood in small quantities. An increased number of these cells may be found in the blood in instances of allergy and infection with intestinal parasites. Additionally, eosinophiles are found in large quantities in nasal mucus in a child who has nasal allergy.

Epiglottis. The "lid" of the trachea, or windpipe.

Epilepsy. A condition of abnormal electrical impulses emanating from the brain which give rise to convulsions.

Epinephrine. See Adrenalin.

Epistaxis. Bloody nose. See page 66 for how to stop a bloody nose.

Erysipalas. A streptococcal infection of the skin no longer frequently seen. In this condition, large areas of the skin become raised, red, and painful; the child may have a high fever and be quite ill. Penicillin is the drug of choice and makes the child well quickly.

Erythema. Abnormal redness of the skin.

Erythroblastosis fetalis. Severe anemia in a newborn infant whose blood has been partially destroyed by antibodies from the mother's bloodstream. Common examples of this condition are found in Rh disease (see Appendix 4) and ABO blood type incompatibility. See page 229.

Erythromycin. An antibiotic frequently used in children to treat respiratory and other kinds of infection.

Ethical drugs. Medicines sold over the counter, that is, without prescription, but not usually promoted to the layman. These drugs are advertised mostly to physicians. See Appendix 2.

Eustachian tube. The tube that supplies air to the middle ear from behind the nose. For a diagram of its location and a discussion of the importance of its proper functioning, see pages 60 and 61.

Exchange transfusion. The process in which all the blood of an individual is changed by removing small quantities of blood and replacing it with fresh blood several times. By the process of dilution the patient's entire volume of blood is changed. This treatment was first devised for newborn infants to exchange the toxic breakdown products of blood that occurred in Rh disease. It has since been adapted for use with older children who have noxious agents in their blood from one of many different causes.

Expectorants. Cough medicines used to lessen mucus. See Appendix 2.

Fainting. Loss of consciousness, usually from some simple cause. Children frequently faint when they have been hurt suddenly, when they have their blood drawn, or when they anticipate some noxious procedure and then relax after the procedure is over and realize they haven't been hurt terribly much. Fainting is of no great significance in children unless it is persistent.

Farsightedness. The ability to see well at a distance but not close up. The medical expression is hyperopia.

Fecal impaction. A state of severe constipation in which the lower rectum is so full that the feces cannot readily be evacuated. This may need to be treated with frequent small enemas of oil or soap suds.

Fetus. An unborn infant, usually after three months after conception.

Fissure, rectal. A split or crack in the skin of the anus, comparable to a split lip. A rectal fissure usually responds to sitting in a tub of lukewarm water three or four times a day and applying a simple healing ointment such as Balmex or Melynor. These ointments should be applied frequently during the day and attempts should be made to push a little ointment into the anal opening.

Fluoride. A chemical that strengthens teeth and retards the formation of dental cavities. It can be added to the water supply or given to infants and children by mouth in small measured quantities daily. Fluoride treatments directly on the teeth are also available at the discretion of your dentist.

Fontanel. A "soft spot" on the head of a newborn infant. It is the location where three or four plates of bone come together but have not yet been joined. There is consequently a "soft spot" between them.

Foreign object. An object that does not belong where it is found. Children have been known to put objects in their eyes, up their noses, and in their mouths, to swallow them, to aspirate them into their respiratory tracts, to put them in their belly buttons, up their penises, in their vaginas, and up their rectums. See page 65 for a discussion of retrieval of foreign objects from the nose. The same technique may be applied to foreign objects in the ear. In most other locations, if they are not readily accessible, they should be seen by your physician.

Frenulum of tongue. The little band of tissue that binds the tongue to the floor of the mouth. It used to be frequent practice to snip this band at birth if the physician thought it was too tight and might result in a "tongue-tied" child. We now realize that no defect of speech occurs as a result of being "tongue-tied," and therefore we no longer snip tongues.

Frostbite. An injury of the skin caused by excessive exposure to cold. The treatment for frostbite is to warm the part involved, quickly but not excessively, to normal body temperature.

Fungus infection. The commonest fungus infection seen in children is athlete's foot. See Appendix 2 for a list of topical medication used for fungus infection. In persistent cases fungus infections may be treated by taking medication internally. This will have to be prescribed by your physician.

Furuncle. A severe abscess with multiple heads or cores which may drain.

Gamma globulin. A part of the blood that contains antibodies that fight infection. Gamma globulin is purified from whole blood and is available to patients exposed to infectious hepatitis or to regular measles if they have not been previously immunized. There are some other specific uses for gamma globulin. However, it is not used in infants and children to fight common upper respiratory infection unless these children are tested and found to have a specific lack of gamma globulin.

Gantrisin. The trade name for a sulfa preparation commonly used to treat urinary-tract and other types of infection.

Genitourinary. Relating to the genital and urinary organs.

Geographic tongue. A tongue that has patches of taste buds alternating with smooth areas, so that it looks like a geographic map in relief.

German measles. Also called three-day measles or rubella. When it afflicts a woman in the first three months of pregnancy, it may cause severe defects in the fetus. All children should be immunized against rubella. See Appendix 1.

G.I. series. An X-ray, or radiographic, study of the upper portion of the gastrointestinal tract. This study usually includes the esophagus, stomach, and small intestine. See Figure 14, page 112.

Glandular fever. Infectious mononucleosis.

Gluten. A substance found in wheat which may cause gastrointestinal disturbances in children who are unable to absorb it. This malabsorption syndrome has been called celiac disease.

Gonorrhea. Of classical significance in pediatrics is the prevention of gonorrhea of the eyes in newborns by means of the Credé procedure, in which a drop of silver nitrate is instilled into the eyes shortly after birth. Sometimes the infant has a purulent discharge from the eyes for a few days following birth. Another complication of the Credé procedure is obstruction of a tear duct, causing simple recurrent discharge from the eye and sometimes excessive tearing. Although these tear ducts may have to be probed later on, most often the obstruction clears spontaneously within the first six months of life.

Grand mal. A type of epilepsy characterized by major generalized convulsions. This will always require care by your physician.

Growing pains. A very real phenomenon occurring at varying times of life and unexplained by medical science. Most commonly the afflicted children awake in the middle of the night and complain of pains of the long bones of their legs. The pains will be real enough to make them cry. They frequently respond to some aspirin, rubbing of the extremity by a parent, and gentle reassurance. These pains have no other medical significance.

Gum boil. Abscess of a tooth, most frequently found in primary or baby teeth. When trauma injures a primary upper front tooth, it may turn dark gray or black. By examining the gum above the tooth after the color has darkened, one may see a pimple develop on the gum surface. This is called a gum boil and represents an abscess of the dead tooth. Gum boils infrequently occur in permanent teeth and to teeth located farther back in the mouth.

Gum cyst. Little bubblelike cyst of clear fluid on the gums of some infants before they develop teeth. They have no clinical significance and usually disappear.

Gynecomastia. The appearance of nubbins of tissue beneath the nipples of adolescent boys. It is very common and may persist for months or years. Not significant in terms of sexuality or disease, it will regress spontaneously in a few years. There is no cause for concern; treatment is reassurance.

Hair ball in stomach. Children who enjoy eating hair and the stuffing from fuzzy animals may develop a mass of hair in the stomach which cannot pass out into the intestines. The condition is very rare.

Hand-foot-mouth syndrome. A condition of small blisters appearing around the hands and feet and in the mouth of some children who are infected by the Coxsackie virus. Its appearance may initially be similar to chicken pox, but these spots do not itch as much, and the disease is not as contagious. No treatment is required; the child invariably gets better.

Harelip. A congenital failure of fusion of the left and right portions of the upper lip, which may extend to and include the lower portion of the nose. It is sometimes associated with cleft palate. Invariably discovered at birth, it is reparable by plastic surgery.

Head lice. Small insects which inhabit the hair and lay eggs, which they firmly attach to the base of the hair. Eggs are called nits. A shampoo is available (Kwell) which will destroy the head lice and loosen the nits so that they can be fine-combed out of the hair.

Heart murmur. An unusual sound heard when listening to the heart. Some murmurs signify heart abnormalities, but many murmurs are of no significance as far as health is concerned, only connoting noisy blood flow.

Heat exhaustion. A type of prostration seen in children especially after vigorous exercise in warm weather. It is usually caused by inadequate replacement of body fluids and salt.

Height. See a discussion of growth problems on page 213.

Hemangioma. A small harmless tumor of blood vessels which makes its appearance at or shortly after birth, reaches its largest size in the first three months of life, and then begins slowly to fade. Ninety-five percent of all hemangiomas disappear completely by age five. Therefore the treatment is observation and nothing more for at least that period of time.

Hematemesis. The medical expression for vomiting blood. Many children who retch violently have streaks of blood in their vomitus. This is due to inflammation of the stomach and esophagus as a result of their forceful retching and has no particular significance.

Hematoma. A collection of blood under the skin, usually caused by trauma. Most hematomas will resolve spontaneously without any difficulty.

Hematuria. The medical expression for blood in the urine. It should always be brought to the attention of your physician.

Hemoglobin. The chemical within the red blood cell that transports oxygen from the lungs to the tissues. For a discussion of the breakdown of hemoglobin as it relates to jaundice, see page 163.

Hemophilia. An inherited bleeding disorder which occurs in males and is transmitted by females. For a discussion of the genetics of this disease and the implications for its future control, see page 228.

Hemophilus influenzae. A bacteria capable of causing severe infection in young children. In its most severe form this infection may cause meningitis or epiglottitis.

Hemoptysis. Coughing up blood. This should always be brought to the attention of your physician.

Hepatitis. An inflammation of the liver. It may be caused by an infectious virus transmitted through the secretions of the mouth and gastrointestinal tract. A person who has been intimately exposed to a patient with infectious hepatitis should receive gamma globulin. One expert has defined those requiring gamma globulin as all the people who have taken meals with the patient in the week prior to the onset of his illness. Another form of hepatitis, known as homologous serum jaundice, is transmitted by the use of unsterilized syringes and needles. This disease has appeared in overwhelming numbers in the past few years as the result of the illegal injection of drugs. This form is called hippie hepatitis.

Hernia. A weakness or opening which allows part of the body to protrude abnormally through that opening. Hernias most commonly occur in children in the umbilical area and in the groin. Most umbilical hernias will close spontaneously in the first few years of life and require no care. Hernias in the groin should be brought to the attention of your physician.

Herpangina. A virus infection of the throat caused by the Coxsackie virus. See pages 78 and 157.

Herpes simplex. A virus that usually causes infection early in life and then may recur sporadically as a cold sore or fever blister near the lower lip. The cold sore runs its course and disappears spontaneously in a week or ten days.

Herpes zoster. A virus that causes shingles. It is thought to be the same virus that causes chicken pox. See page 154.

Hexachlorophene. A chemical found in certain soaps used to prevent or treat skin infection. For many years hexachlorophene was used in the routine bathing of infants in nurseries and has cut the incidence of infection. However, recent evidence indicates that hexachlorophene may appear in unusually high amounts in the brains of infant monkeys similarly bathed, and its indiscriminate use has been discontinued. Nevertheless, it is still a good cleansing soap, especially useful for injured and infected areas, and for this purpose its use has not been discontinued.

Hiccups. A spasmodic repetitive sharp intake of breath thought to be due to irritation of the diaphragm. There are many lay maneuvers to cure hiccups; they are all as good or as bad as anything we physicians can come up with, and therefore should be tried if they are not too drastic.

Hip, congenital dislocation. Found mostly in female infants.

The hip joint is abnormally formed, and the upper portion of the thigh may be dislocated high on the pelvis. This will always require the diagnosis and treatment of your physician.

Hives. A raised, itchy eruption of the skin, usually an allergic reaction and readily treatable in most instances with anti-histamines.

Hoarseness. A coarseness and thickening of the voice caused by irritation or inflammation of the vocal cords in the voice box. See Figure 11, page 90.

Hookworm infection. A parasitic infection commonly found in the Southern states and due to the invasion of human bare feet by the hookworm, which inhabits the soil. This infection will always require the care of your physician.

Hormones. Chemicals secreted by endocrine glands which play important roles in varying functions in the human body. Examples of hormones are insulin, which is required for the metabolism of sugar, and growth hormone.

Humidity. For a discussion on the necessity of adequate humidification in upper respiratory infection, see page 79.

Hydrocele. An accumulation of clear liquid in the sac surrounding the testicle. A common finding in newborn infants, it most often disappears without treatment. However, hydroceles are frequently associated with inguinal hernias and should therefore be observed carefully.

Hydrocephalus. Obstruction of the normal flow of cerebrospinal fluid out of the head causes its enlargement. This condition usually comes on after birth and will be detected by the regular checkups provided most newborn infants.

Hydronephrosis. A condition in which the kidney enlarges because of obstruction somewhere along its outflow tract. It may also be associated with chronic infection.

Hydrophobia. An old term for rabies.

Hyperopia. Farsightedness.

Hypertension. High blood pressure. This condition can occur in children for a number of reasons, but all of them are rare.

Hyperthyroidism. Overactivity of the thyroid gland.

Hypothyroidism. Underactivity of the thyroid gland.

Hypoxia. Inadequate oxygen reaching the tissues.

Immunization. The process by which one confers immunity by giving small doses of an antigen or noxious substance in order to have the patient build up appropriate antibodies to that substance.

Impaction, Fecal. See Fecal impaction.

Impediment, Speech. See Frenulum of tongue.

Incontinence. Inability to control the outflow of feces or urine.

Incubation period. The period of time between the acquisition of the infecting agent of an impending infection and the development of symptoms of that infection.

Incubator. A mechanical device for keeping objects warm. In childhood illness it most frequently applies to the enclosure that keeps premature infants warm and isolates them from the outside world.

Infantile paralysis. Poliomyelitis. For adequate protection against this dread disease, see Appendix 1.

Infectious mononucleosis. A viral infection, usually seen in older children, characterized by fever, extreme sore throat, malaise, and excessive feeling of tiredness. This condition may be misdiagnosed originally as acute sore throat, perhaps streptococcal in origin. Actually the streptococcus is present in the throat in 20 to 40 percent of all cases. Mononucleosis requires the attention of your physician.

Inflammation. A condition in which a portion of the body has an increase in the number and size of blood vessels, is usually painful and tender, and may be warm to the touch. Infection may or may not be present.

Influenza, Viral. Upper respiratory viral disease characterized by fever, upper respiratory symptoms, cough, malaise, headache, and weakness.

Influenzae, Hemophilus. See Hemophilus influenzae.

Ingrown toenail. This condition usually occurs on the great toe of either foot; it may occur on either side and is usually caused by improper growth of a nail into the fleshy substance. The toe then usually becomes infected. It will respond to hot soaks and removal of the offending portion of the ingrown nail.

Inguinal hernia. A hernia found in the groin. The portion that herniates in boys is usually a small piece of intestine, and it appears on the abdominal wall. Later in life it may appear in the scrotal sac. In girls the part that herniates is frequently the ovary and almost always appears on the abdominal wall.

Injections. See Appendix 1.

Inoculation. Injection. See Appendix 1.

Insect bites. Generally divided into two types: the stinging insects and the nonstinging insects whose bite is merely troublesome. These latter bites should be kept clean and will usually disappear without great difficulty. If itching becomes a problem, local applications of calamine lotion may be used, and the oral administration of antihistamine drugs may be helpful. See also Bee stings.

Insulin. The hormone, secreted by the pancreas, that is essential for metabolism of sugar. In patients with diabetes, insulin secretion is inadequate and must be supplemented with insulin given by injection.

Intrauterine infection. Infection that enters the uterus and may infect the fetus. One example is rubella (German measles). Women whose membranes have ruptured more than twenty-four hours prior to delivery are watched very carefully to see if their infants become ill shortly after birth.

Intravenous feeding. A method of feeding fluids and chemicals directly into the veins of a child who is dehydrated. This procedure is always carried out in a hospital.

Intussusception. A condition occurring at times in young children in which a portion of their intestine telescopes on itself and becomes stuck. This child will begin to complain of sporadic cramp abdominal pain and then develop signs of intestinal obstruction.

Iron. A nutrient required in adequate amounts for blood formation. It frequently requires supplementation, especially under one year of age.

Itching, medicine for. See Appendix 2.

Itching, rectal. See Pinworm, p. 125.

IVP. Abbreviation of intravenous pyelogram, X rays of the kidneys.

Jock itch. A fungus infection of the genital area in males, which is most frequently seen in the summertime and among athletic young men. It may be treated locally with antifungal medication. See Appendix 2.

Joint pains. Most significant in pediatric patients suspected of having acute rheumatic fever or juvenile rheumatoid arthritis. They are not to be confused with growing pains, which occur in long bones rather than in joints. See Growing pains.

Kaopectate. A kaolin-pectin mixture frequently used to treat diarrhea. See Appendix 2. There is a concentrated form of Kaopectate called Kaocon, which is more palatable to younger patients because it is flavored; the dose may be halved.

Knock-knee. A congenital abnormality seen in many children, frequently related to flat feet.

Koplik spots. Little white spots surrounded by a red area in the mucous membrane of the mouth of infants and children about to develop the rash of regular measles. With the advent of adequate immunization, this phenomenon should become extinct. See Appendix 1.

Kwell. Used in the treatment of head lice and pubic, or crab, lice.

Kyphosis. An abnormal curvature of the upper portion of the spine.

Labia. Greek for "lips." Commonly used to denote the outer-most folds of the genital area in females.

Laryngitis. An inflammation of the larynx, usually causing hoarseness, and frequently in children heralding the onset of croup.

Laryngotracheobronchitis. An inflammation or infection of the respiratory tract. It is usually caused by a virus and begins in the larynx with hoarseness, progresses to the trachea with barking cough, and culminates in the bronchi, where the cough may become more productive of mucus.

Laxative. Drug used to facilitate bowel movements.

Leukemia. Cancer of the white blood cells.

Leukocytes. White blood cells. Their main function is to fight infection.

Lice. The plural of louse. An insect that may inhabit head hair, pubic hair, eyelashes, and eyebrows. See Head lice; Crab lice.

Lip blister in newborns. A common occurrence in vigorously suckling newborns. It is of no medical significance and will disappear.

Liquiprin. An aspirin substitute. See Appendix 2.

Lisping. A speech impediment. Not related to tongue-tie.

Lockjaw. Tetanus. See Appendix 1.

Lye poisoning. Lye is a caustic agent. When poisoned with lye, one should *not* be made to vomit. Consult your physician immediately.

Malabsorption. Inadequate absorption of foodstuffs and nutrients in the gastrointestinal tract. For an example of this, see Celiac disease; Gluten.

Malocclusion. Improper clenching of the teeth, usually due to poor dental alignment. The dental specialist who treats this condition is called an orthodontist.

Mastitis. Inflammation of the breast. It may occur in small infants and/or their mothers.

Mastoiditis. Inflammation in the mastoid bone, usually resulting from infection, and almost always secondary to chronic middle-ear infection.

Measles, German. See German measles.

Measles, regular. Rubeola. This disease is characterized by fever and cough of varying degrees which may last for several days. There follows the outward appearance of upper respiratory infection and, finally, the development of a red spotty rash. Regular measles is avoidable! Adequate immunization is available and should be given to all children at one year of age. See Appendix 1.

Meconium. A thick black sticky substance which is found in the gastrointestinal tract of newborns prior to milk feeding. They evacuate this substance within the first few days of life.

Medicines. See Appendix 2.

Membrane, mucous. The lining of almost any cavity of the human body which communicates with the outside world and which secretes mucus.

Membrane, Tympanic. The eardrum.

Meningitis. An inflammation, usually an infection of the meninges, which are the membranes surrounding the spinal cord and extending up into the head. This disease is characterized by fever, irritability, sleepiness or vomiting, and a stiff neck. It must be treated quickly and strenuously in the hospital. It will always require the attention of your physician.

Metatarsus varus. An inward curvature of the foot. Although this deformity will frequently straighten out by itself, it is readily correctible with orthopedic shoes or casts.

Middle-ear infection. Otitis media. The common ear infection frequently associated with colds in toddlers and young children. See page 68.

Migraine headache. This type of headache occurs in children as well as adults. Its symptoms may be different from the classical headache in adults, but in a migraine-headache-prone family, any kind of severe recurrent headache associated with any other kind of recurrent abnormal behavior should be considered a migraine possibility.

Miliaria. A rash comprised of multiple tiny white-headed pimples seen most commonly over the face, neck, and shoulders in infants who are overdressed. The treatment is less vigorous bundling. Also called prickly heat.

Mittelschmerz. Abdominal pain noted in some postpubertal girls or women occurring midway in their menstrual cycle between one period and the next. This is thought to represent a small amount of bleeding into the abdominal cavity when an ovum pops off the ovary and begins its journey down the fallopian tube.

Mold. An allergen frequently found in damp places, mold is the basis for allergic symptoms in many children in the middle of the winter.

Molding of the head. The newborn head is malleable so that its shape can be changed if necessary when passing through the birth canal. Immediately after birth, many newborns' heads are distorted and misshapen. They round up beautifully in a few days.

Mole. Also called a nevus, this is a brown "beauty spot" that may appear on any individual at any time. Only the very dark bluish-black ones require the attention of your physician.

Molloscum contagiosum. Single small white firm pimples whose centers contain a pearly hard mass. Mollosca occur singly and then multiply into aggregations of pimples of varying sizes. They may spread (thereby the name) and are known to be caused by a virus. Treatment will require the help of your physician: it is reasonably simple.

Mongolism. A chromosomal abnormality which may have one or several characteristics, but mental retardation is almost always one of them. The medical term is Down's syndrome or trisomy 21. This disease will usually be diagnosed at birth.

Monilia. An infection caused by the organism *Candida albicans,* appearing as thrush of the mouth, monilia dermatitis, or diaper rash in many newborns. See pages 165 and 174.

Mononucleosis, infectious. See Infectious mononucleosis.

Mosquito bite. Superficial red raised bump that appears following the bite of a mosquito. It itches, but can be treated simply with calamine lotion and meticulous attention to cleanliness.

Motion sickness. Nausea and upset stomach associated with riding in a moving vehicle. It can occur as the result of riding in a car, boat, airplane, or one of the rides in a carnival. The best treatment is prevention, but if this is not possible, certain drugs are available which alleviate it. See Appendix 2.

Multiple sclerosis. Most commonly an adult disease, multiple sclerosis may appear in children. A degenerative disease of the nervous system, the first symptom is apt to be difficulty in vision. The type of visual difficulty is rapid loss of vision, almost total but usually transitory. This disease will always require the attention of your physician. Fortunately, it is very, very rare.

Mumps. See Parotitis.

Murmur, heart or cardiac. See Heart murmur.

Muscular dystrophy. Unfortunately, this disease usually occurs in children. Its onset is described as slow and steady progressive weakness, frequently associated with, paradoxically, enlargement of the calf muscles so that they look quite muscular. This is a *very* rare disease.

Mycosis. Fungus infection. See Appendix 2.

Mycostatin. A trade name for nystatin, a drug used predominantly to treat monilia infections. It is available on prescription to treat thrush and thrush diaper rash.

Myopia. Nearsightedness.

Nail infections. Infections that completely surround the nail bed are called onychiae; when they appear on only one side of the nail bed, they are called paronychiae. Sometimes they can be treated with the frequent application of hot soaks, but most often they will require the attention of your physician. It's worth trying yourself, however.

Narcotics. Addictive drugs whose dispensation is controlled by the federal government and requires a license from the Bureau of Dangerous Drugs and Narcotics.

Nausea. The feeling of upset stomach and a desire to vomit.

Navel. The belly button. The medical term is umbilicus.

Nearsightedness. Myopia, the inability to see objects at a distance.

Neo-Synephrine. A decongestant medication usually found as nose drops; an oral preparation is also available. See Appendix 2.

Nephritis. An inflammation of the kidneys. The commonest type in pediatrics is acute glomerulonephritis, an uncommon disease which follows streptococcal infection.

Nephrosis. A kidney disease similar to nephritis but whose course is much more chronic and whose prognosis is not quite as good. This disease is characterized by a lessening of the amount of urine being produced and the accumulation of body fluids. This results in swelling of various parts of the body.

Newborn. An infant is considered newborn during the first month of life.

Nervous habits. Sometimes called tics. Some examples of tics are eye blinking, sighing, coughing, and stuttering. The best treatment for these nervous habits is to ignore them.

Nightmares, and pinworm. Frequently a child who awakes with nightmares an hour or so after being in bed is suffering from pinworms.

Nipples, in infants. Infants' nipples sometimes secrete a drop or two of a white substance which has been called witches' milk. This has no significance and will disappear within a few days.

Nits. The eggs of lice which are attached to the root of hairs. See Lice.

Node, Lymph. A gland in the lymphatic system which may be found in varying locations throughout the body. They have a tendency to enlarge in the presence of infection.

Ob-gyn. An abbreviation for obstetrician-gynecologist, a physician who treats the special problems of women and delivers their babies.

Obstetrician. A medical specialist who practices obstetrics, the management of childbirth cases.

Oculist. A physician who specializes in diseases of the eye. A synonym is ophthalmologist.

Omphalitis. Inflammation or infection of the navel in a newborn.

Ophthalmologist. See Oculist.

Optometrist. A nonphysician specialist who prescribes glasses and also teaches optometric exercises to help cure certain visual problems.

Oral polio vaccine. A vaccine given by mouth which is capable of preventing poliomyelitis. It is also known as Sabin vaccine. See Appendix 1.

Orthodontist. A dentist who specializes in the straightening of misaligned teeth.

Orthopedist. A physician who specializes in bone problems in children and adults.

Orthoptic training. A method, utilizing visual exercises, to aid in certain visual functional defects.

Osgood-Schlatter's disease. A condition that occurs in adolescents in which the tibial tubercle, the bump below the front of the knee, swells and becomes painful. This disease is quite common and is as well known to athletic trainers and coaches as it is to physicians. It requires no specific treatment, will remain for months to years, and then disappear.

Ovulation. The process of an ovum or egg popping off the ovary midway in the menstrual cycle. See Mittelschmerz.

Palate, Cleft. See Cleft palate.

Palsy, Cerebral. See Cerebral palsy.

Paralysis, infantile. See Infantile paralysis.

Paregoric. A drug, usually purchasable in small quantities over the counter, which is useful in slowing down bowel action and treating diarrhea.

Paronychia. See Nail infections.

Parotitis. Inflammation and swelling of the parotid gland, located in front of, beneath, and behind the earlobe. Epidemic parotitis is the medical term for mumps. See Appendix 1 for a vaccine which can prevent mumps. Parotitis may occur in recurrent form in older children. It usually responds to antibiotics.

Pediatrician. A physician who specializes in the treatment of children.

Pediculosis. Infestation with lice.

Penicillin. An antibacterial drug which has been useful in the treatment of many childhood diseases, most especially streptococcal infections. It requires a prescription.

Penis, in diaper rash. It frequently happens that a diaper rash will be associated with a specific sore at the very tip of the penis. This is called a meatal ulcer. It usually responds to a bland ointment. If diapers are particularly rough, a diaper liner may be used.

Perforation of eardrum. The draining of a middle-ear infection or abscess by natural means. Most eardrum perforations in children heal up quickly with adequate treatment and do not necessarily recur or stay perforated. It is only chronic perforations, long-standing ones, or ones that result from long-standing disease that may debilitate a person permanently. And yet, newer techniques make even many of these reparable.

Peritonitis. Inflammation, usually infection, of the peritoneum, the sac that encloses the abdominal contents. Peritonitis, a complication of perforation of the appendix, used to be a dread disease, but is reasonably well handled now with the proper antibiotics and surgery.

Pertussis. Whooping cough. Pertussis is hardly ever seen in infants any more because of adequate immunization. However, it does crop up in some teen-agers who have not had their immunity boosted in many years. It is a pesky disease but not a dangerous one as it may be in infants. Your physician can treat it.

Petit mal. A type of convulsion or seizure disorder in which the patient loses consciousness only very briefly, for seconds at a time, but possibly many times a day. The child does not usually fall over or undergo any severe spasmodic manifestation. Rather, he seems to stop what he is doing, briefly hesitate for a few seconds, and then resume normal function. Episodes such as these should be brought to the attention of your physician.

Pharyngitis. Sore throat.

Phenobarbitol. A drug, usually a sedative. However, in certain children phenobarbitol has a paradoxical reaction; it stimulates rather than sedates.

Phenylketonuria. Synonyms for this inherited disorder are PKU and phenylpyruvic-oligophrenia. This disease, most commonly seen in blond, blue-eyed babies, is one of inadequate enzyme action which may result in mental retardation. All infants in the United States are now tested for this disease at birth. It is very rare, approximately one case in forty thousand births being reported, and can usually be treated by diet if caught early.

Phimosis. The condition in which the foreskin of the penis cannot be retracted back behind the head of the penis. Phimosis is normal in infants. Later in life the foreskin becomes retractable in most instances.

Phobia. A medical expression meaning "fear of."

Phototherapy. A form of therapy used in the treatment of jaundice in newborns.

Pica. The eating of abnormal substances. Children who eat paint and plaster from broken walls can be said to have pica.

Pill, the. The birth control pill, a female hormone which if taken according to directions will prevent pregnancy.

Pink eye. Conjunctivitis.

Pityriasis alba. White patches that occur on the face in children. Frequently mistaken for fungus infection. These patches may come and go for years, but eventually disappear. Their cause is not known.

Pityriasis rosea. A virus infection in which a specific rash appears and persists for approximately six weeks. This condition will always require diagnosis by your physician but will not require treatment.

PKU. See Phenylketonuria.

Placenta. A fleshy umbrellalike organ that resides in the womb, or uterus, and from which the infant receives nourishment during pregnancy through the umbilical cord. After birth, the placenta is discarded.

Plantar warts. Warty growths that occur on the sole of the foot. They are particularly troublesome because they grow in instead of out. Two over-the-counter medications which may be helpful in treating plantar warts are Freezone and Compound W.

Pleurisy. Inflammation of the pleura, or lining around the lung. Fluid may accumulate in the chest.

Pleurodynia. One-sided chest pain associated with a Coxsackie virus infection.

Pneumothorax. A small perforation in the lung which allows that lung to collapse and free air to move out into the chest cavity.

Poliomyelitis. See Infantile paralysis.

Pollenosis. The state of being allergic to pollen.

Polyp, nasal. A condition, rare in children, frequently associated with allergy, in which mucous membrane cysts occur in the nasal cavity. They frequently require removal.

Port wine birthmark. A type of birthmark, usually extensive, which may occur on any area of the body and which resembles a port wine stain.

Postmaturity. An infant may remain in the uterus for too long, that is, more than forty weeks. It may become malnourished because the placenta may lose some of its ability to function. These infants have long fingernails, they have lost weight, and they may have unusually wrinkled skin.

Pox, Rickettsial. A rare, contagious viral infection, similar to Rocky Mountain spotted fever, and transmitted by a small insect called the mouse mite. It begins with a single pimple, which turns black and scales, and is then followed by fever and a blistery-like rash. Your physician should be consulted.

PPD. An abbreviation for purified protein derivative. This substance is used to test one's reaction to tuberculin protein. It is similar to the tuberculin tine test. See Appendix 2.

Prednisone. A pure form of synthetic adrenal hormone used as a medication.

Premature infant. An infant born before nine months' gestation is completed. Premature infants frequently need to be kept in the hospital for a while. They are usually kept in incubators.

Prescription. An order for medication written out by a physician and given to a pharmacist for preparation. See Appendix 2 for a list of medications obtainable at the drugstore without prescription.

Prickly Heat. See Miliaria.

Prolapse of the rectum. A condition in which a portion of the mucous membrane of the rectum becomes detached from its underlying attachment and protrudes from the rectum. Fortunately, this condition is rare.

Psoriasis. A skin condition characterized by patches of scaling and flaking of the skin. It is rare in children, but when it occurs, it's apt to be on the scalp. In adults it is more frequently seen on the back of the elbows and the front of the knees.

Psychiatrist. A physician who specializes in diseases of the mind.

Psychologist. A doctor of psychology who specializes in normal and abnormal human behavior.

Ptomaine poisoning. Food poisoning.

Puberty. The time of life when a child undergoes hormonal changes which produce typical maturation into adulthood.

Pumice stone. A stone used as an abrasive to wear down horny or very hard callous tissue. It may be used for warts.

Purpura. Abnormal bleeding into the skin.

Purulent. Productive of pus.

Pus. The liquid breakdown product of infection. A thick, yellow, often foul material composed of bacteria, white blood cells, and tissue debris. Accumulations of pus should be drained.

Pustule. A small pimple which contains pus.

Pyelitis. Inflammation, and usually infection, of the main urine-collecting areas of the kidney.

Pyelonephritis. Inflammation and infection of the entire kidney.

Pyloric stenosis. A condition usually occurring days or weeks after birth, most commonly in a firstborn male child, in which the outflow valve of the stomach becomes large and over-muscled. The opening of the valve is thereby diminished in size, and stomach contents cannot readily pass through and into the intestines. The infant vomits in a projectile fashion, does not gain weight, and requires surgery for the alleviation of his symptoms.

Pyrexia. Fever.

Pyuria. Pus in the urine.

Quarantine. The isolation of individuals afflicted with contagious disease. Sometimes the isolation of individuals who are potentially infected with contagious disease until it has been shown that they do not have such an infection. There are only a very few diseases that require quarantine at the present time.

Rabies. A dread infectious disease transmitted by the bite of an infected mammal. Most domestic animals, especially pets, are well protected against rabies by inoculations. Most of the rabies in the United States occurs in small wild animals such as foxes, wild dogs, bats, skunks, mice, and rats. Any child who has been bitten by a wild animal, *without that animal having been provoked into the biting,* and especially if that animal has seemed to be acting in a peculiar manner, should be seen by a physician. If possible, and with the greatest of precautions, the animal should be trapped so that it can be sacrificed and examined. Fortunately, rabies is rare.

Rectal suppositories. Commonly used in the treatment of constipation. However, rectal suppositories may contain different medications to treat different diseases. For example, aspirin suppositories are available over the counter to use in children who are vomiting. Suppositories are also available through prescription to treat asthma, nausea, and vomiting, to provide sedation, and for many other uses.

Red blood cells. The cells in the blood that contain hemoglobin, which carries oxygen throughout the body.

Regurgitation. A little vomiting.

Retardation, mental. An abnormal lack of intelligence.

Rh factor. See page 229 and Appendix 4.

Rickets. A deficiency disease characterized by bowing of the legs, prominences of the sternum, and swelling of the ends of the long bones. Due to inadequate vitamin D, rickets is almost never seen nowadays.

Rickettsial pox. See Pox, rickettsial.

Ringworm. A fungus infection of the skin. See Appendix 2 for a list of topical antifungal medications. Some ringworm is difficult to treat and may require internal medication on prescription from your physician.

Ritalin. A psychotherapeutic drug similar to Dexedrine, which has been used to quiet excessive activity in "hyperactive" children. It has also been recommended for the treatment of certain behavior problems and school problems in children. This drug needs your physician's prescription.

Rocky Mountain spotted fever. A rare disease, transmitted by the bite of a tick, seen nowadays throughout the temperate climates, especially in North America. It will require the diagnosis and treatment of your physician.

Rose fever. Pollenosis occurring in the spring.

Rubella. See German measles.

Rubeola. See Measles, regular.

Rupture. See Hernia.

Sabin polio vaccine. See Oral polio vaccine.

St. Vitus's dance. See Chorea.

Salk polio vaccine. The first vaccine developed to provide prevention against poliomyelitis. This vaccine required injection in an initial series and boosting every year or so. It has been replaced by the Sabin oral polio vaccine.

Salmonella infection. A bacterial infection which produces diarrhea and fever. Typhoid is a type of salmonella infection. Readily treated with modern antibiotics.

Scabies. A condition in which a tiny insect burrows under the skin and sets up a fierce itching and allergic reaction.

Scarlatina. Mild scarlet fever.

Scoliosis. A curvature of the spine from left to right or vice versa.

Scrotum. The bag beneath the penis that contains the testicles.

Scurvy. A deficiency disease due to lack of vitamin C (ascorbic acid). It is very rare in the United States at the present time.

Seasickness. A form of motion sickness associated with traveling on a boat. See Appendix 2 for a medication that may alleviate this problem.

Seat worm. See Pinworm.

Seborrhea. A condition of excessive oiliness occurring mostly on the face and scalp. It may be similar to eczema or dandruff. One good medication for seborrhea of the scalp is a shampoo called Sebulex.

Sedatives. Drugs that sedate, or calm down.

Sedimentation rate. A blood test sometimes used to determine whether or not there is inflammatory activity going on in the body. Inflammatory activity is found in many infectious diseases and certain rheumatic disorders. It is a nonspecific test.

Seizure. A convulsion.

Sepsis. Blood poisoning.

Shigella infection. A severe bacterial infection frequently occurring in children. Symptoms are high fever and diarrhea. Readily treated with antibiotics.

Shock. See Cardiovascular collapse.

Sickle-cell anemia. A problem in abnormal hemoglobin formation leading to distorted red blood cells. This disease is found chiefly in blacks.

Sleeping sickness. See Encephalitis.

Smallpox. See Appendix 1.

Smegma. A secretion found normally under the foreskin in males and in the folds of the labia in females.

Snake bites. Uncommon and not usually poisonous. Snake bites require the immediate attention of your physician if a poisonous snake is suspected.

Soft spot. See Fontanel.

Spasm, muscular. See Charley horse.

Spastic paralysis. A type of paralysis in which the muscles are contracted and tight, rather than limp. Seen in children with cerebral palsy.

Speed. An amphetamine.

Spermatozoa. Sperm. The male sex cell, supplied with a tail, which when injected into the female combines with the ovum to form the beginning of the new human being.

Spinal curvature. See Scoliosis.

Spinal meningitis. See Meningitis.

Spitting up. Simple regurgitation or mild vomiting.

Squint. Strabismus.

Stammering. A speech impediment similar to, but not precisely, stuttering.

Staphylococcal infection. The staphylococcus is a bacteria frequently found in purulent infections. This organism is capable of becoming resistant to a number of antibiotics, including penicillin. For this reason it has achieved a bad reputation in hospital-acquired infections. However, infection acquired by most outpatients (that is, out of the hospital) is readily treatable.

Steroids. The chemical classification of adrenal hormones, i.e., cortisone.

Stomatitis. Inflammation or infection of the mouth, usually associated with viral infection and frequently due to an infection with the herpes or Coxsackie virus.

Strawberry mark. See Hemangioma.

Stridor. Excessive and abnormal sounds are made in the act of breathing. This condition is usually seen in infants and small toddlers as a result of immature structures in the back of the mouth, throat, and upper respiratory tree. Stridor may also be associated with croup or foreign bodies in the upper respiratory tract. Stridor should be brought to the attention of your physician if it is serious or debilitating.

Stuttering. A speech impediment characterized by frequent repetition of parts of words; frequently considered a tic, or nervous habit.

Sty. An abscess of a gland on the eyelid.

Sun lamp. A good treatment for acne, especially in winter.

Tear ducts. Little ducts located inside the corner of the eye, which drain tears down into the nose. Tear ducts in the newborn may become obstructed by the chemical conjunctivitis that occurs as the result of the instillation of silver nitrate.

Testicle. One of two egg-shaped globular structures hanging in the scrotum beneath the penis. The site of sperm production.

Testis. Testicle.

Tetanus. A bacterial infection associated with dirty wounds which is quite severe and has a high mortality rate. Tetanus need not occur in appropriately immunized individuals. On the other hand, the use of booster immunizations against tetanus has been too frequent. See the official recommendation for tetanus immunization and boosters in Appendix 1.

Tetracycline. A broad-spectrum antibiotic. It has fallen into disuse in pediatric patients because of its proven ability to stain teeth. However, there are times when its use is indicated, even in small children. It requires a prescription.

Thrombocytopenia. A condition in which there is a diminution in the number of platelets in the circulating bloodstream. Platelets are necessary in the process of blood clotting. The disease therefore is sometimes manifested by improper clotting of blood or a hemorrhagic process. The medical synonym is idiopathic thrombocytopenic purpura (ITP). This condition will always require the care of your physician.

Thyroid gland. An endocrine gland located in the neck (not to be confused with the thymus gland) which, under the direction of the pituitary gland, secretes thyroid hormone into the bloodstream to regulate metabolic and physical activity within the body. The simplest symptom to remember for underactivity of the thyroid gland (hypothyroidism) is underactivity of the patient. Conversely, the simplest symptom associated with overactivity of the gland (hyperthyroidism) is overactivity of the patient. Disorders of the thyroid gland will always require the care of your physician.

Tic. See Nervous habits.

Tick. A small insect capable of transmitting Rocky Mountain spotted fever. Usually found on long-haired animals.

Tine test. A screening test used to detect tuberculosis. For a routine of tuberculin tine testing, see Appendix 1.

Tinea. Ringworm: a classification of fungus organisms capable of causing infection in man.

Tongue-tied. See Frenulum of tongue.

Tonsillectomy. The operation performed for the removal of tonsils.

Tonsillitis. Inflammation, usually infection, of the tonsils.

Toxemia of mother. A condition that may occur in the last trimester of pregnancy, in which the mother develops hypertension. Early delivery of the infant may be necessary.

Toxoid, tetanus. A booster injection of tetanus. The indications for tetanus boosters may be found in Appendix 1.

Toxoplasmosis. An infection caused by the protozoa *Toxoplasma gondii,* which when acquired in childhood or adult life is of no apparent clinical significance and has no symptoms. However, when a woman acquires toxoplasma infection during pregnancy, it may be transmitted to the unborn fetus and cause serious disease. Toxoplasma infection in newborn infants will always require careful study, diagnosis, and treatment by your physician.

Trachea. The windpipe.

Trenchmouth. Stomatitis, or infection of the mouth. This disease may require the attention of your physician or dentist if it is severe. Otherwise, frequent mouthwashes and gargles (one-third hydrogen peroxide to two-thirds warm water) will be helpful.

Tylenol. Acetaminophen, an aspirin substitute.

Tympanic membrane. The eardrum.

Typhoid fever. Infection with the organism *Salmonella typhosa,* characterized by fever and diarrhea. This disease will require the attention of your physician.

Ulcer. An erosion of a surface on or within the body. To the layman, ulcers usually mean erosion of the mucous membrane lining of the stomach. When an ulcer occurs in an area that is liberally supplied with blood vessels, bleeding frequently occurs. Stomach ulcers are usually thought to be an adult disease, but can occur in children of all ages, albeit rarely.

Ulcerative colitis. See Colitis, ulcerative.

Umbilicus. The belly button, or navel.

Unconsciousness. An abnormal state of not being aware of

one's surroundings. This is one of the cardinal danger signs of illness in a child.

Undernourished child. A condition found in lower socioeconomic groups within the United States, but very rare in the majority of suburban children.

Undescended testicle. The testicle does not accomplish its normal descent into the scrotum prior to birth. Surgery may be required for correction.

Ureter. The tube that connects the kidney with the urinary bladder.

Urethra. The tube that connects the urinary bladder with the outside world.

Urinary bladder. Collects and holds urine prior to its elimination from the body.

Urologist. A surgical specialist; a physician who is knowledgeable in the treatment of problems of the urinary tract.

Urticaria. Hives. Actually, a histamine reaction of the skin. Raised elongated streaky swellings, usually white and surrounded by a reddened area. Itches intensely.

Uterus. The womb.

Vaccination. Strictly speaking, the process of immunizing a person against smallpox with vaccine. Actually, this expression has come to mean immunization against any disease.

Vaccinia. A generalized eruption that sometimes occurs in association with smallpox vaccination. The eruption may consist of intensely itchy pimples, or multiple small vaccination reactions. Any rash that occurs with a smallpox vaccination should be seen by your physician.

Vaginal discharge. Except in the newborn, any vaginal discharge that occurs in the prepubertal female child should be brought to the attention of your physician. Infection or a foreign body within the vagina is possible. During and after puberty, vaginal discharge should be considered as in the adult. Minimal discharge requires no treatment; excessive or foul discharge should be investigated.

Vaporizer. A mechanical device for increasing humidity in overheated homes. There are hot steam vaporizers and cold vaporizers. The hot ones have the advantage of creating particles of smaller size which are capable of going farther down the respiratory tree. Cold vaporizers have the advantage of being safer. Your physician should be consulted for help in making the decision about which would be more appropriate in your situation.

Varicella. Chicken pox.

Varicocele. An accumulation of dilated veins, seen in some adolescent boys, in the scrotum. It does not seem to bother them but may become troublesome in later life and require surgery.

Variola. Smallpox.

Verruca. Wart.

Vertigo. True dizziness (when the room actually seems to spin around, not when the patient just feels lightheaded).

Viral hepatitis. See Hepatitis.

Volvulus. A twisting or knotting of one or more loops of intestine, which may cause intestinal obstruction.

Wall eye. Strabismus in which one of the eyes assumes an outward position.

Warts. Small growths, thought to be caused by a virus, which appear on various parts of the body and which are troublesome but never serious. Plantar warts (occurring on the soles of the feet) are particularly troublesome because they hurt when the patient walks, and the pressure of his walking makes them grow in rather than out. Warts may be variously treated; they may be worn down with a pumice stone, or they may be treated with compounds such as Freezone or Compound W. These are mild acid solutions and frequently cure them. See page 190.

Wheezing. The patient has difficulty with the expiratory, or breathing-out, phase of the respiratory cycle. There is partial obstruction due to spasm of the bronchi. See page 102.

White blood cells. Leukocytes. Cells important in combating infection.

Whiteheads. Pimples with little white heads, commonly seen in acne. Also in newborn infants as miliaria, or prickly heat.

Whooping cough. See Pertussis.

Witches' milk. See Nipples, in infants.

Worms. See Pinworms.

Wry neck. A spasm or Charley horse of one of the muscles of the neck. The head is tilted to one side; any movement from this position is quite painful. The medical expression is torticollis.

X ray. A method of making images of the inside of the body by means of radiation. X rays may be helpful in the diagnosis of disease. They should never be used indiscriminately in children, in whom the effect of radiation may have more consequences than in the adult.

Xyphoid. The tiny bone at the bottom of the sternum (breast plate).

Yellow fever. A tropical disease seen infrequently in the United States. For patients going to areas endemic with yellow fever, prophylactic immunizations are available.

APPENDIXES

Appendix 1.

*Immunization: How, When, Why,
and Reactions*

Diphtheria/Tetanus/Pertussis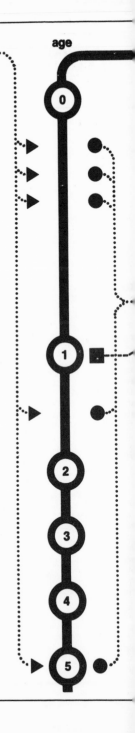
Whooping Cough

(D/T/P)

This immunization is given as a series of three injections (each containing small amounts of the vaccine against all three diseases). They begin at one or two months of age and are spaced at one or two month intervals until all three injections are given. This is the initial series.

A reaction may occur, consisting of fever, fussiness, irritability, soreness, swelling or tenderness of the injection site. This should not last longer than forty-eight hours.

Boosters at eighteen months and five years of age.

Diphtheria/Tetanus (D/T)

After the age of five years, (see D/T/P above) boosters against Diphtheria and Tetanus are recommended every ten years. Thus the first booster of D/T should be given at about fifteen years of age.

The same reaction may occur as is described above for D/T/P. Note that the Pertussis fraction has been left out; for older children, Whooping Cough no longer constitutes the threat that it did in infancy. On the other hand, the reaction rate of the Pertussis fraction of the vaccine increases with age. Thus the continued administration of Pertussis component becomes unwise and unnecessary.

Tetanus Boosters

If a child's immunization series is current, that is, if the schedule described above under D/T/P and D/T has been maintained, NO additional Tetanus boosters are recommended unless the wound is considered "contaminated". To me, this means wounds that are inflicted under filthy circumstances and are very difficult to clean, or wounds which become infected. When a wound is considered "contaminated", a Tetanus booster should be given if the child has not had one within the past *five years*.

This is quite a change from the old rule which required a tetanus booster if the patient hadn't had one within the past year. We have known for a long time that too much tetanus was being given. However, old habits are hard to break, especially when the disease is such a dangerous one, (the mortality rate of Tetanus is still 50%) and the shot is considered so innocuous.

On the other hand, recent evidence indicates that Tetanus occurs only in unimmunized individuals, or people who have not had boosters in ten to thirty years. In addition, some investigators are beginning to question the possible deleterious long-term effects of too many doses of Tetanus. Finally, a gamma globulin preparation is now available which is loaded with Tetanus antibodies, and which has been found to be highly effective in treating early Tetanus cases. I believe the new recommendation is valid and welcome.

Immunization schedule

Measles/Mumps/Rubella
German Measles

(M/M/R) tm Merck, Sharp & Dohme

Protection against all three of the above "common contagious diseases of childhood" may now be obtained in a single injection. It is given once, at one year of age or later, (it should *not* be given earlier) and will not require a booster. As far as is now known, it will provide lifelong immunity to all three diseases. Single components and combination vaccines are also available for children who have been immunized to any of the single diseases.

The measles component may cause a reaction consisting of mild fever, cough, or minimal rash five to twelve days after the injection. The rubella component may cause aching joints in adolescents or older patients in ten to twenty-one days. This is transient and should not be disabling. Reactions are not usually seen to the mumps component.

Sabin Vaccine
Poliomyelitis—"Polio"

This is a vaccine administered by mouth as two drops of "medicine" and provides lifelong immunity against poliomyelitis ("polio"). No reaction is expected. It is given at the same time as the D/T/P; three doses in the first six months of life, and boosters at eighteen months and five years.

Smallpox Vaccination

Discontinued! This vaccination has finally been judged to be no longer necessary. The risk of morbidity (illness) and even mortality (death) that may be associated with vaccination is now considered far greater than that of the disease. (There has been no smallpox in the United States since 1949!) And the risk of importation of smallpox is so minimal (because the disease is being so well controlled worldwide) that it is not worth the risk of vaccination.

N.B. Overseas travelers may still have to be vaccinated, depending upon their destinations. These regulations are in a state of flux at the time of this writing, and so specifics cannot be given.

The Tuberculin Test

The tuberculin test is not an immunization, but rather an intradermal (*in* the skin) injection which tests for the presence of tuberculosis. It replaces the old "patch" test, and even replaces the chest X-ray as a screening test for tuberculosis in children and adults who have never been tested before, or whose reaction to the tuberculin test has always been negative. However, once the test produces a positive reaction, it remains positive thereafter, and an annual chest X-ray is *mandatory*.

The presence of a positive tuberculin test does not mean that a child has tuberculosis. Rather it means that the tuberculosis germ has entered his body, and that a defense mechanism has been set up to combat tuberculous infection. Our defense mechanisms usually win the battle, and most children with positive tuberculin reactions do not have clinical tuberculosis, and will not go on to develop this dread disease. However, a few will not be so lucky, and it is these few for whom the annual skin test is important.

The first test should be done late in the first year, and *prior* to the Triple Virus Vaccine (see opposite). After that, I believe it should be done annually, throughout adolescence. The purpose of the test is to identify children who have converted their tuberculin reaction from negative to positive *within the first year of their conversion*. These are the children who are most likely to develop clinical tuberculosis, (albeit the likelihood is quite remote) and also the children in whom clinical tuberculosis is most likely to be prevented by starting them promptly on medication.

Appendix 2.

Useful Over-the-Counter Drugs and Doses

The following drugs are sold over the counter in pharmacies. They do not require the prescription of your physician. (This may vary somewhat from state to state.) In many instances they are equal in potency and usefulness to prescription drugs, and always cheaper. This is because the pharmacist does not have to keep careful records of their sale, like prescription drugs.

Many of them are called "ethical" drugs—that is, they are advertised and promoted to the medical profession, but not to the public. I have found it useful to tell my patients about them, and feel that they are safe and helpful when used according to the directions on the label.

Doses appearing on the label are usually small and safe. When the recommended dose varies according to the weight of the child, it should be followed exactly. However, frequently the dose is given by age group, and then some adjustment should be made for the very large or very small child. It is often recommended that the physician be consulted ,regarding dosage instructions for the child less than three years of age. I have found it safe to use two thirds of the three-year-old's dose for the two-year-old, and one third of the three-year-old's dose for the one-year-old. I agree that for children less than one year of age, the physician should be consulted.

Aspirin substitutes (*acetaminophen*). Useful to reduce fever and relieve pain, especially in children allergic to or intolerant of aspirin. Also advantageous because a liquid preparation is available, they do not promote a bleeding tendency, and there are no known cases of overdosage or toxicity. Available as:

Liquiprin
Tempra
Tylenol

Nosedrops (*phenylephrine*). For congested, blocked, and stuffy noses, usually associated with simple upper respiratory infections. May also help liquefy thicker nasal secretions, and will reduce inflammation causing recurrent nosebleeds. Use ⅛% for infants under one year and ¼% for older children. Do not use ½ or 1%. Available as:

Neo-Synephrine
Biomydrin

Decongestants. To decongest the head, *not* the chest. Useful mostly in colds and more complicated *upper* respiratory infections, especially in children prone to middle-ear infections. If there is an allergic history (patient or family), use with an antihistamine.

Pure decongestants
Sudafed elixir and tablets

Neo-Synephrine elixir
Decongestants with antihistamine
  Triaminic syrup
  Novahistine elixir

Cough medicine. Before selecting a cough medicine for your child, try to figure out what kind of a cough he has and why he has it. Then you can more intelligently decide what you want the cough medicine to do. (Obviously we want all coughs to "go away," but sometimes they are useful in cleaning out the respiratory tract and should persist awhile.) Coughs can be considered "wet" or "dry" depending upon how much mucus you hear rattling around. The mucus can sometimes be identified as coming from down in the chest, or up in the nose and throat area. And coughs can occur mostly at night, mostly during the day, or around the clock.

Dry coughs that occur only in the morning and seem better after breakfast are usually due to low humidity and dry, irritated mucous membranes. Get out the vaporizer. When a dry cough comes on after the child goes to bed, and then seems to become mucous after a while, this frequently means that the child is draining nasal and sinus cavities because of a change of position. These coughs should be treated with decongestants during the day to try to keep the mucus from accumulating, and may require suppressants at night to let the child get to sleep. However, if a child has a history of sinusitis, it may be better to withhold the decongestants so that the mucus doesn't get too thick and viscous. Nose drops will be helpful here. Sometimes these coughs persist into the daytime, and are then associated with postnasal drip. Decongestants are helpful here too.

When dry coughs occur intermittently day and night, especially when they are associated with fever, it usually means that the child is coming down with a respiratory infection. These coughs may need suppressant at night, but should be treated with expectorants during the day, because mucus is almost sure to follow, and when it does, it should be kept loose. Possibly the driest, tightest cough we see is the one associated with the sudden onset of croup (see Chapter 3). Expectorants are most helpful here too. Rarely, a dry, sudden-onset cough will appear immediately following a choking episode, most often in a large infant or toddler. This cough is incessant and persistent, not associated with fever, and seems to severely harass the child. It should be brought to the attention of your physician at a relatively early stage as it may mean that a foreign object (usually food) has been inhaled into the respiratory tract.

If your child has a constipation problem, suppressant cough medicines should be used with special care. These preparations all contain codeinelike substances, which are quite constipating. Of course, this is even more true in prescription cough suppressants, which contain true codeine.

Coughs that are loose and juicy and seem to come from the lower chest almost always mean that mucus is being produced. These coughs require expectorants to keep the mucus thin and allow it to be brought up. Most children don't actually expectorate (spit out the mucus) but swallow it. This is good enough since it is being eliminated from the other end of the gastrointestinal tract. Occasionally so much mucus is produced that the child becomes nauseated and vomits. Mucus may then be seen in the vomitus, and expectorants should be discontinued for a while, unless the child can be encouraged to spit out his mucus. In addition, even wet coughs may have to be suppressed at night in order to allow the child to get his rest.

Since it has been noted that allergy plays such a significant role in upper and lower respiratory infection, antihistamines have been included in many ethical cough preparations. They are helpful in children producing lots of mucus from the nose and sinus area and who are known to be allergic. However, they should *not* be used when one suspects there is mucus in the *lower* respiratory tract, or when there is wheezing. Antihistamines have a tendency to decongest or dry mucus in the chest, making it thicker, more viscous and therefore more difficult to move. Expectorants are indicated here to keep the mucus loose. In addition, your physician may want to prescribe specific medication for the wheezing.

Pure expectorants
  Robitussin
  2G
  Ipsatol
Expectorant plus decongestant
  Robitussin-PE
Expectorant plus decongestant plus antihistamine
  Triaminic expectorant
Suppressants
  Cheracol D (includes an expectorant)
  Novahistine-DH (includes decongestant and antihistamine)
  Novahistine Expectorant (includes decongestant, antihistamine, and expectorant)
  Dorcol (includes decongestant and expectorant)

Pure Antihistamines
  Allerest
  Allertoc

Diarrheal Medicines. These have been subdivided into plain "thick mixtures" and those with drugs to slow down bowel action. In many states, small amounts of paregoric may be obtained without prescription.

Pure thick mixture

    Kaopectate (unflavored)

    Kaocon (concentrated Kaopectate—advantageous because only half the dose is required, and it is flavored)

Pure antispasmodic

    Paregoric

The dose for paregoric is not apt to be on the label. Use one teaspoonful in a little fruit juice for an adult-sized child, and proportionately less by weight for smaller children. It should not be repeated more often than every four hours, and should be replaced by a call to your physician if abdominal pain persists after two doses.

    Combination (thick and antispasmodic) mixtures.

    Donnagel

    Parepectolin

Laxatives. Here again you need to analyze what you're trying to do. Some children are too busy or too lazy to have complete evacuation of their bowels and need stimulation. Others who eat little fruit or bulk produce dry stools which need softening by having water added to them (stool softeners). And children with dry stools, and especially children who are in the habit of retaining their stools, need lubrication. Remember that laxatives are habit-forming, and should never take the place of a diet that will promote good bowel habits. Fruit and vegetables provide bulk for stools; among the fruits, prunes (and prune juice), dates, figs, raisins, and apricots are especially helpful. Bran cereals also help, and if the child has candy, make it licorice. Lubricants are mostly mineral oil, and should be given only at night, since this substance may interfere with the absorption of fat-soluble vitamins. And oils should never be force-fed. If fats or oils get into the lungs, there's trouble.

Lubricants
  Mineral oil (pure)
  Neocultol (flavored)
Stimulants
  Milk of Magnesia
  Castoria
  Ex-Lax
Stool softeners
  Colace
Combinations
  Haley's M-O (milk of magnesia and oil)
  Peri-Colace (stool softener and stimulant)

Motion Sickness and Antinausea Drugs. Remember that if nausea and vomiting are associated with abdominal pain in a child who does *not* have diarrhea, your physician ought to know about it.

Dramamine
Bonine
Marezine

Skin Preparations. There are literally thousands of them on the market. A professor of pharmacology used to tell us to learn about a few of them, depending upon what we wanted them to accomplish, and forget all the others. Stop shopping!

Diaper rash (soothing and protective)
  Vaseline
  A and D ointment

Desitin (not Desenex!)

Diaper rash (healing)

   Balmex

   Melynor

Anti-itch (see antihistamines and aspirin)

   Calamine lotion

   Calagesic ointment

Lubricants

   Vaseline

   Mineral oil

Cleansing soaps—antibacterial

   Phisohex (should not be used for total body scrubs of newborn infants)

   Dial

   Safeguard

Antibacterial preparations (usually may be obtained in creams, lotions, ointments, and powders)

Neosporin

   Neo-Polycin

   Caldesene (also anti-fungal)

Antifungal preparations (usually may be obtained in creams, lotions, ointments, and powders)

   Tinactin

   Desenex (not Desitin!)

   Caldesene (also antibacterial)

Acne preparations (usually available as soaps and creams. Remember that nothing replaces the washcloth and hot water, at least three times per day!)

   Fostex

   Phiso-Ac

Eczema (this preparation works better if it is applied very frequently—up to six times per day—or not at all)

   Tarbonis—2-ounce tube and one-pound jar.

Cradle cap and dandruff (remember that nothing replaces vigorous massage of the scalp, even in infants and
even directly over the "soft spot." I've never seen an infant
injured yet!)

Sebulex

Appendix 3.

Growth Charts

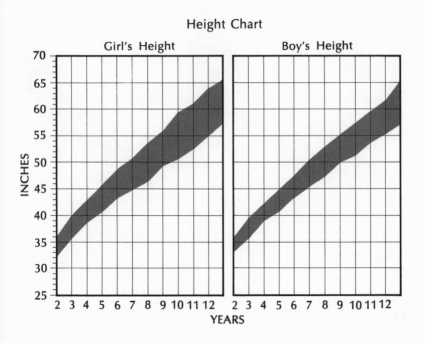

Height Chart

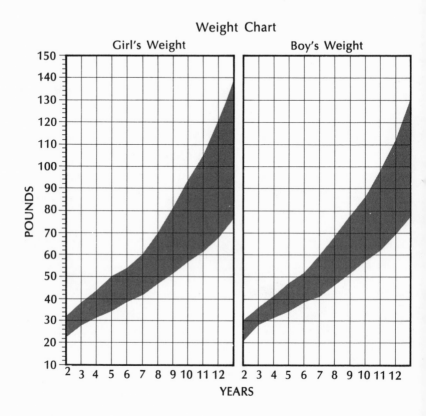

Appendix 4.

The Genetics of Rh Disease

All human cells (except sex cells, i.e., sperm and ova), have twenty-three *pairs* of chromosomes within their nuclei, for a total of forty-six chromosomes. Sex cells have twenty-three *individual* chromosomes (*not* pairs). Therefore, when two sex cells unite, twenty-three new *pairs* of chromosomes result in a new nucleus of the first cell of a new human being.

Chromosomes contain *genes,* which are protein bits of information that determine the physical characteristics of the individual. One such pair of genes determines whether that individual will contain Rh substance on his red blood cells, and therefore be Rh *positive,* or lack this substance and be Rh *negative*.

Since the gene that determines the presence or absence of the Rh factor is a dominant one, if either gene of the pair is an Rh positive gene, the person will be Rh positive. Conversely, in order for an individual to be Rh negative, *both* genes must be negative for the Rh factor.

The Genetics of Rh Disease

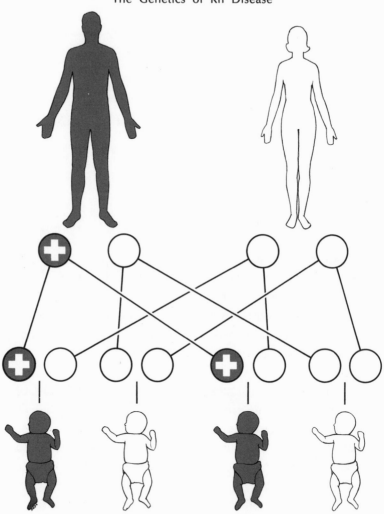

Heterozygous Male (positive)

The Genetics of Rh Disease

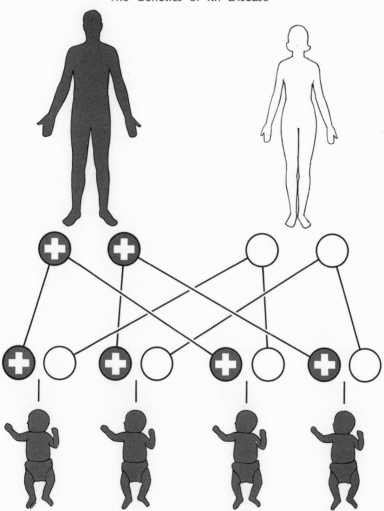

Homozygous Male (positive)

In order for Rh disease to occur in an infant, his mother must be Rh negative and his father Rh positive. However, the father may be *heterozygous* (Rh factor positive on only *one* gene) or *homozygous* (Rh factor positive on *both* genes). The diagrams illustrate how a homozygous Rh positive father will have *all* Rh positive children, whereas with a heterozygous Rh positive father, each child has a fifty percent chance of being Rh positive.

Index

Abdomen (*See also* specific conditions): newborn, 167-68; pain in, 109-33

ABO incompatibility, 235

Abortion, 231-32

Abscesses, 186, 235-36. *See also* Teeth; etc.

Acid (LSD), 236

Acidosis, 236

Acne, 187-89, 236, 303

Achromycin, 236

Activity in sickness, 46-47

Adenitis, 236

Adenoids (adenoidal tissue), 60, 61, 63, 85-87, 160, 236

Adeno-pharyngeal-conjunctival fever, 160

Adenovirus, 237

Adrenalin, 237

Age groups: and allergies, 137-42; and behavior, 28; growth charts, 305-6

Air cleaners, 145

Airsickness, 237

Albumin in urine, 237

Allergies, 134-52, 300 (*See also* specific substances, symptoms); age groups and, 137-42; environmental control, 144-46; fallacies, 147-49; home treatment and allergists, 150-52; methods of contact, 134-36; rational approach to, 141-44

Alopecia, 237

Alveoli, 97, 98, 99

Amblyopia, 237

Ammonia(cal) dermatitis, 173, 237

Amniocentesis, 231, 237

Amphetamines, 238

Ampicillin, 238

Anemia, 238. *See also* specific types

Animals (pets): allergies, 146; bites, 238; and poison ivy, 179

Anorexia, 238

Antibacterial preparations, 303

Antibiotics, 36-37, 238. *See also* specific uses

Antibodies, in infection, 55, Rh, 229, 230

Antifungal medicine, 238-39, 303

Antihistamines, 239, 300. *See also* specific uses

Anti-itch medicine, 303

Antinausea drugs, 302

Antipyretics, 239

Anus, itching of. *See* Pinworm

Aphasia, 239

Appendicitis, 111-13, 126-27

Appendix shown, 112

Appetite, loss of (anorexia), 238

Arthritis, 239

Ascorbic acid, 239

Asian flu, 239

Aspirin, 44-45, 49 (*See also* specific uses); substitutes, 297; suppositories, 39

Asthma, 103, 151